PEDIATRICS BOARD REVIEW® QUESTIONS & HOT TOPICS

• 100% Money Back Pass Guarantee •

Your Certification SYSTEM for Passing the Pediatric Boards

• MASSIVE Online Community •
• Board-Focused, Manageable Content •
• Powerful Mnemonics •

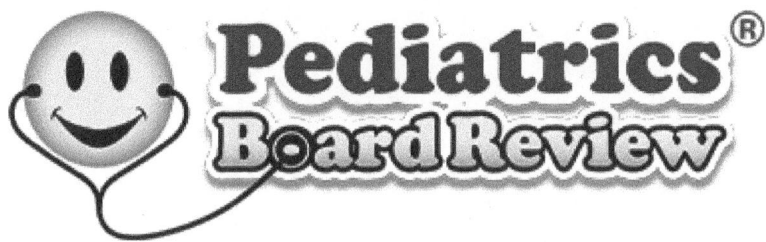

EFFICIENT LEARNING So You Can Enjoy Life & Have More Fun!

Written by Ashish Goyal, MD

www.PediatricsBoardReview.com

COPYRIGHT INFORMATION

© 2025 Pediatrics Board Review, Inc.

All rights reserved. No part of this document may be reproduced or transmitted in any form or by any means, electronic, mechanical, photocopying, recording, digital storage or otherwise, without prior written permission of Pediatrics Board Review, Inc.

Any reproduction, presentation, distribution, transmission, or commercial use of the concepts, strategies, methods, materials, and all other trademarks, copyrights, and other intellectual property owned by Pediatrics Board Review, Inc. in any media, now known or hereafter invented, is prohibited without the express written permission of Pediatrics Board Review, Inc. It is prohibited to use any device, now existing or hereafter invented, to make an audio and/or visual recording, transmission, or broadcast of any online, offline, audio, or video materials of Pediatrics Board Review, Inc.

The legal entity "Pediatrics Board Review, Inc." may be referred to as "Pediatrics Board Review" or "PBR."

Reproduction of Pediatrics Board Review, Inc. material without written permission is punishable by law.

ISBN: 978-1-300-62682-4

INTRODUCTION TO THE "EASY" PBR EXPERIENCE! (Read This!!!)

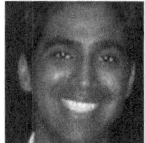 Hi there! I'm Ashish Goyal, the author and creator of Pediatrics Board Review (PBR). I've had the privilege of guiding thousands of pediatricians through their board exams. As a double-boarded physician living on a remote landmass, I've seen my work impact pediatricians nationwide.

More than just study materials, PBR is a system designed to **limit overwhelm, give clear direction, and maximize efficiency**. You'll be given the **essential information** needed to ace the boards, without all of fluff. The results speak for themselves and demonstrate that PBR is ideal for **first-timer test-takers and those who are at high risk of failing**.

The key to our success has been the **PBR Certification System**. The system is built around **clear and concise information and guidance**. The concise information is available in both **hardcopy and digital formats**, and the guidance tells you exactly how to use the resources, and wehen. All you have to is follow the checklist.

This **multimodal and formulaid approach** has not only been shown to **enhance learning and retention**, but it also places a **strong emphasis on test-taking strategies**—a focus I've been pioneering for over a decade to achieve seemingly impossible results, such as helping **one pediatrician who passed on his 10th attempt and another pediatrician finally find success on her 11th attempt**.

PBR is the ONLY pediatric review to offer this approach. It was created for first-time test-takers to help them pass easily, but has made miracles happen for those who have previously failed.

Our knowledge base resources include a Core Study Guide, a Q&A book, online editions of our books, an audio course, a video course, and a Virtual Atlas of Pediatric Pictures. Information is **presented in the same order** so your efforts are maximized for efficiency.

Our "success accelerator" resources include live ASK THE EXPERT webinars, ASK THE EXPERT question portals for every chapter in the Core Study Guide, Personalized Study Schedules created for you by Team PBR, Blueprints for Success based on your risk profile, an Online Test-Taking Strategies Course, a Live Test-Taking Strategies & Deep Study Course, a private online community, and much more.

PBR is tailored for a wide range of needs – from **residents** needing to increase ITE scores to **first-time ABP exam** takers to, to **repeat test-takers**, to pediatricians preparing for the **recertification exams** and those in need of **CME/MOC credits**.

More than just study materials, PBR is an **integrated system** offering **content, test-taking skills, personal guidance**, and **passionate community support** to help you **cement knowledge and surpass your expectations**. Our alumni's success demonstrates that **our system is all you need** to pass your exams.

PBR's first-time pass rate for the ABP initial certification exam is estimated at **98%**, which is significantly higher than the national average of **81-84%**.

In short, Team PBR and I aim to help you *get* board certified and *stay* board certified. We're passionate about what we do, and we're always here to help. Please reach out if you need anything along your journey!

All the best,

Ashish & Team PBR

WHAT CHALLENGES IS PBR SYSTEM SOLVING FOR YOU?

EFFICIENCY THROUGH SYSTEMS AND INNOVATION

Most board review books and courses simply hand you a book and say, "good luck." That's how I studied for the USMLE exams, the pediatric board exam (twice) and the internal medicine board exam. **I was completely isolated!** After purchasing thousands of dollars of board materials, I was left to go through the books and video courses with no real guidance, no feedback from my peers, and absolutely no advice from the authors (besides a one-page preface).

NO MORE ISOLATION

Because of how excruciatingly painful that was, **I've created a community of pediatricians for you to study with and a blueprint** of what to study, how to study it and how to do so **EFFICIENTLY**!

GUIDED TO SUCCEED

ALL of PBR's resources are created with your *time* in mind. I've aimed to solve these questions over the years:

* Will the resource be **easy to use**?
* Will it provide **more value** than existing resources AND provide that value in a **more streamlined** fashion?
* Can we make the resource **easily accessible via smartphones and tablets**?
* Will the resource **reinforce the core concepts** laid out in the PBR and in the Q&A book **instead of overwhelming** you with new concepts?
* Can we make the resource **portable** (e.g., audio or video?) so that it can be used at times when a physician, or a mom, or a dad, or a gym-enthusiast, would not normally be able to study?
* Can we teach you how to **become a better studier** and maximize your time in front of the books **through Deep Study**?
* Can we assist by creating Personalized Study Schedules for you that **map out your study time**?
* Can we help you **become a better test-taker** through courses on test-taking strategy?
* Can we create **an easy-to-follow formula for success**?

PBR is a <u>system</u> unlike anything you have ever experience before in your medical career. The Core Study Guide is written in easy-to-understand language and provides you with hundreds of time-saving memory aids. The online systems allow for one-click access to hundreds of high-yield images across the web. The Q&A book has some of the highest yield and most board-relevant questions available.

You also have a ready-made study group of hundreds of pediatricians to help you EFFICIENTLY blow past trouble spots in your studying. Plus, your questions, requests for clarification, and submissions of potential errors are all used to create a Corrections & Clarifications Guide that is released annually to the entire PBR community right before the initial certification exam to give you a boost in your knowledge base and understanding of the materials.

All of these efficiency-focused systems **SAVE YOU OVER 100 HOURS OF TIME** and give you **flexibility in your life to enjoy your family, your friends, or to reinvest that time** into repetition of the PBR material.

A critical component of ANY individualized board review plan is to go through the study material MULTIPLE times. **PBR is concise, makes the learning manageable,** and will allow you to feel confident on your test day because of well-prepared you are for your exam.

WHAT IS THE BEST BUNDLE FOR ME?

→ PGY1 – PGY2 (IN-TRAINING EXAM PREPARATION)

Your main goal should be exposure to board-relevant content. I recommend that you either get the **Ultimate Bundle Pack + MP3 Bundle** or the **ALL ACCESS PASS**. If you want to sign up for multiple years to ensure access through the date of your exam, email us to get a big discount. For group discounts, visit www.pbrlinks.com/GROUPS.

→ INITIAL CERTIFICATION EXAM PREPARATION (PGY3 & HIGHER)

In general, the **NO BRAINER** and the **VIP BUNDLE** are the best bundles. The No Brainer is the one that most low-risk initial certification exam takers enroll into. It gives you everything you need to develop your fund of knowledge while also providing our introductory Online Test-Taking Strategies Course to help you learn test-taking strategies. You also get up to three 90-Day Personalized Study Schedules created for you by Team PBR.

→ WHAT IS YOUR RISK PROFILE? IF YOU DON'T KNOW... YOU COULD BE IN TROUBLE.

Your plan of attack MUST be based on how likely you are to pass or fail. What is your risk profile? If you don't know, please visit www.pbrlinks.com/RISK-CALCULATOR immediately and find out.

For **LOW-RISK** test-takers, the **ALL ACCESS PASS** is also a very good option. It focuses on a multimodal learning experience to develop your fund of knowledge and gives you access to our ASK THE EXPERT live webinars and online question portals. This bundle does not focus on test-taking strategy, and it only offers one 90-Day Personalized Schedule. The assumption is that you tend to do very well on exams, you've never failed any medical board exam, and you are very good with time management.

For **MODERATE-RISK** test-takers, the **NO BRAINER** or the **VIP BUNDLE** would be the bundles to choose from. The No Brainer includes the All Access Pass, the Online Test-Taking Strategies Course, and it also offers three Personalized Study Schedules created by Team PBR. **However**, this exam is not like any other medical board exam you have taken, and implementing the teachings and strategies from the VIP Bundle (discussed below) will ensure that you pass! So, it's my belief that the "insurance" is worth it.

For **HIGH-RISK** test-takers, the **VIP BUNDLE** is the right choice. It includes the No Brainer and a seat in one of our Live Test-Taking Strategies & Deep Study Courses. These courses help you with advanced test-taking strategies and allows you to break through the plateau that you will reach if you only use our Online Test-Taking Strategies Course. The Deep Study lectures are often called "life changing" because they help you become a MUCH better manager of your time, your energy, your life's priorities, and your focus. The VIP BUNDLE also includes Group Deep Dive calls to help you understand PBR's best practices and to help you break through barriers during your board prep.

→ MOCA-PEDS ASSESSMENT QUESTIONS

You **do not** need the PBR Core Study Guide and Q&A Book. They are good supportive resources, but we have a very inexpensive **MOCA-PBR Study Guide & Test Companion** that is specifically created to help you pass your quarterly questions. Every year, we create 1-page topic summaries to cover ALL of the ABP Learning Objectives and Featured Readings for General Pediatrics in concise, 3-page summaries. If we do our job right, you will pass without needing to study anything else!

→ MOC EXAM (4-HOUR, PROCTORED RECERTIFICATION EXAM)

This is a smaller, easier version of the initial certification exam. For most board-certified pediatricians, the **Ultimate Bundle Pack + MP3 Bundle** or the **ALL ACCESS PASS** are sufficient. If you are someone who has struggled with standardized exams in the past, then you should enroll into the **NO BRAINER** bundle.

WHAT ARE THE 7+ RESOURCES THAT YOU HAVE ACCESS TO?

The <u>**ALL ACCESS PASS**</u> and the <u>**NO BRAINER**</u> are by far the most popular memberships for anyone taking the initial certification board exam. If you have one of these, **please make sure you take advantage of <u>all</u> of these resources!** If you are at moderate or high risk of failing, please also read the previous page because the <u>VIP Bundle</u> might be the right one for you!

1. **PBR'S COMMUNITY!** This includes Ashish Goyal, "Team PBR," PBR's summertime webinar content experts, and the **MEMBERS-ONLY DISCORD GROUP**. <u>JOIN THE INVITE-ONLY DISCORD GROUP NOW</u>! <u>Do not study in isolation</u>! You have a community of pediatricians to support you. **The COMMUNITY aspect is one of the most valuable components of the PBR system**. Studying for a board exam can be GRUELING, but having others to lean on for clarification, advice or just some moral support can make all the difference in your studying experience. Just have a look!

PRIOR PRIVATE COMMUNITY COMMENTS FROM BEFORE WE RECENTLY SWITCHED TO DISCORD

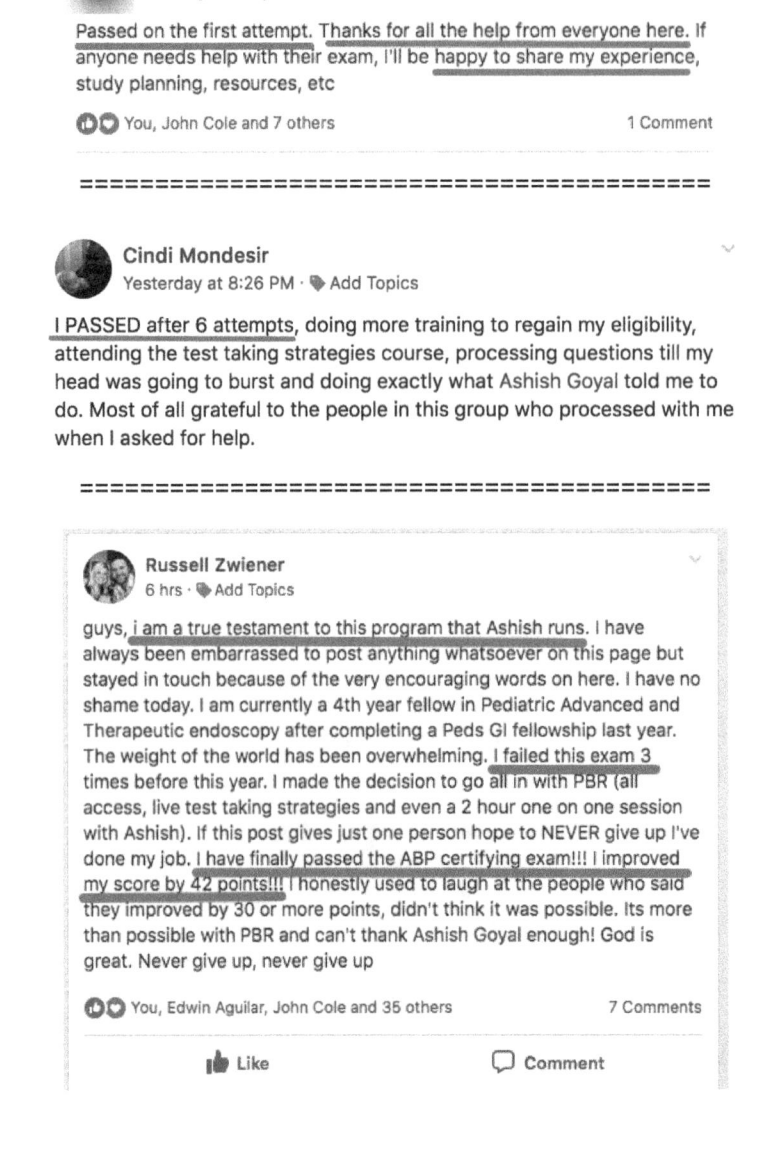

Reza
5 hrs · Add Topics

Passed on the first attempt. Thanks for all the help from everyone here. If anyone needs help with their exam, I'll be happy to share my experience, study planning, resources, etc

You, John Cole and 7 others — 1 Comment

===

Cindi Mondesir
Yesterday at 8:26 PM · Add Topics

I PASSED after 6 attempts, doing more training to regain my eligibility, attending the test taking strategies course, processing questions till my head was going to burst and doing exactly what Ashish Goyal told me to do. Most of all grateful to the people in this group who processed with me when I asked for help.

===

Russell Zwiener
6 hrs · Add Topics

guys, i am a true testament to this program that Ashish runs. I have always been embarrassed to post anything whatsoever on this page but stayed in touch because of the very encouraging words on here. I have no shame today. I am currently a 4th year fellow in Pediatric Advanced and Therapeutic endoscopy after completing a Peds GI fellowship last year. The weight of the world has been overwhelming. I failed this exam 3 times before this year. I made the decision to go all in with PBR (all access, live test taking strategies and even a 2 hour one on one session with Ashish). If this post gives just one person hope to NEVER give up I've done my job. I have finally passed the ABP certifying exam!!! I improved my score by 42 points!!! I honestly used to laugh at the people who said they improved by 30 or more points, didn't think it was possible. Its more than possible with PBR and can't thank Ashish Goyal enough! God is great. Never give up, never give up

You, Edwin Aguilar, John Cole and 35 others — 7 Comments

👍 Like   💬 Comment

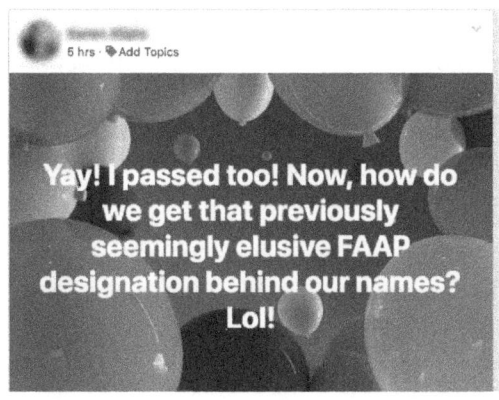

==

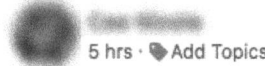

5 hrs · Add Topics

I PASSED!!!! I failed three times then found out that my job would only allow me to take it one more time before letting me go. And if that wasn't stressful enough I found out I was pregnant. Studying with a full time job, 3 kids and one on the way was awful but I pushed through. I took that test 37 weeks pregnant and thankfully my baby held tight. Finally I thank god I'm able to say I am board certified. Thank you PBR #wonthedoit

You, John Cole and 25 others   7 Comments

==

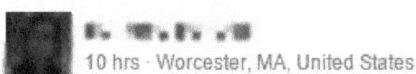

10 hrs · Worcester, MA, United States

Made it!!! Thank you Ashish, PBR staff and Facebook crew for your help and support with the Boards!!!

==

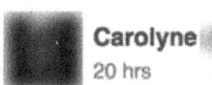

Carolyne
20 hrs

Passed! Thank you Ashish and PBR crew!

Visit the following link to join our community: www.pbrlinks.com/community

2. **HARDCOPY PBR CORE STUDY GUIDE**: YOU WILL LOVE YOUR "PBR!" It is at the center of your success blueprint. Carry it everywhere, highlight it, draw pictures, create mnemonics and add notes to help you cement the 2500+ MUST-KNOW topics in this book. After your exam, I promise you that you will MISS IT!

3. **HARDCOPY PBR Q&A BOOK**: KNOW this book! It is NOT a random collection of questions. The material should be considered CORE material for you to study over and over again. Carry it around and mark it up! Make sure you review this book as many times as you review the Core Study Guide.

4. **ONLINE VERSIONS OF THE PBR CORE STUDY GUIDE**: All 2500+ topics are available in a scrolling PDF style format and in a topic-by-topic, **searchable** format. Keep this open and use the **one-click**

image links while you study or after each two-hour block of studying. It's **iPhone/smartphone compatible, iPad/tablet compatible and desktop compatible**.

5. **ONLINE VERSION OF THE PBR Q&A BOOK**: Have a few minutes while at work? Open the scrolling PDF version of the Q&A book and go through one or two questions.

6. **PBR WEBSITE**: The website has a TREMENDOUS amount of valuable content. Each article was written to help address a need expressed by pediatricians. Read as many of the articles as you can! There is also a TOOLS section where you can find links to <u>discounted pediatric board review question banks</u>.

7. **PBR'S TEST-TAKING STRATEGIES**: Physicians are not taught HOW to take tests. **GOOD pediatricians with sound clinical reasoning WRONGLY believe that** a board exam is a measure of one's knowledge base, and thus a measure of one's abilities as a clinician. That is completely false.

Exams require mastery of the English language, mastery of pacing, mastery of your emotional state during an exam, and an understanding of the **deceptive tactics** employed by question-writers to create **seemingly possible yet blatantly WRONG answer choices**.

PBR's <u>ONLINE TEST-TAKING STRATEGIES & COACHING COURSE</u> (included in the No Brainer bundle) offers **insights into this "board game."** You will stop viewing question as miniature patients and start viewing them as miniature riddles. Riddles with concrete rules and strategies to help you reach the correct answer quickly (**even when you often lack the clinical knowledge!**). Understanding the rules of the game will completely change your outlook on how to prepare for the exam and how to use board review questions for PRACTICE instead of content. **I HIGHLY recommend the PBR Test-Taking Strategies & Coaching Course for anyone who is taking the boards, but especially for those who are "at risk." This includes you if:**

- You have failed this exam at least once
- You typically score below the national average on your board exam scores
- You have failed ANY USMLE Step exam
- You were classified as "at risk" during residency based on your in-training exam scores
- You are more than 1 year out of residency

The course helps you understand the <u>techniques and skills</u> associated with answering board-style questions correctly. **We've helped MANY pediatricians finally pass the boards after failing multiple times, including ONE, TWO, THREE, FOUR, FIVE, SIX, SEVEN, NINE, and TEN times!** So, helping you should be easy.

To get just a taste of how you can increase your board scores immediately, and to learn a few of the rules to the "board game," click here and read a PBR article I wrote titled, "*3 Strategies to Skyrocket Your Score!*" - www.pediatricsboardreview.com/techniques

Also, visit **www.pediatricsboardreview.com/strategy** and watch a FREE test-taking strategies session right now.

TEST-TAKING STRATEGY COURSE MEMBER TESTIMONIALS
(FROM MEMBERS OF OUR ONLINE COURSE AND/OR OUR LIVE COURSE)

*Ashish, I did it. I can't thank you enough for creating an amazing system to keep me on track with my studying. And the $2000 for the **live weekend** test taking course was well worth it. Doing the technique during the test kept me focused and allowed me to eliminate wrong answers. Thank you for all the great advice, sticking to the material, memorize, memorize, memorize then practice practice practice. **After 4 failed attempts**, it was exhilirating to finally read the words, "we are PLEASED to announce you PASSED!"   I will definitely recommend your program. God Bless*

- Dr. Yessenia Castro-Caballero, Board Certified Pediatrician

---

I believe I broke the record taking this test 10 times!!!! I finally passed on the 10th... I appreciate sincerely all your help, I have cried cried all day today, after too many years and thousands of dollars spent, finally this is in the past now. Thank you so much.

- Dr. Pablo Chagoya

---

*I PASSED finally!!!!!!!!!!!!!! So relieved and it's all because of you!! I would not have done it without the **live courses**... Thank you Ashish!!! You are the best!!*

Frannie
Your devoted PBR fan :)

- Dr. Frances Liu, Board-Certified Pediatrician who **increased her score by 18 points after failing 3 times**

Definitely helped to get a better understanding of the "board game" that Ashish mentions. **I'm sure I've fallen prey to those traps in the past.**

Also, knowing the types of questions and the algorithm to figuring out how to spend my time answering the questions-- never would have thought about the Hybrid approach to just reading the last line of the vignette for "this/these" questions.

Really didn't know that I shouldn't be spending time reading through the whole vignette... or doing the "top to bottom" approach!

Overall it was great and I really appreciate you taking the time and effort putting this together and making sure that we can succeed our first time around.

Helped immensely with reading/understanding the "English" of the questions - **I actually would've gotten one example question wrong in the past had I not used the AaCNI mnemonic**

I had very little time to prepare for the boards... The core study guide helped me focus on topics that were high yield on the exam. In addition, **the strategies taught by Ashish were very helpful and is what I believe helped me PASS**. I would highly recommend the PBR for anyone needed to review in a short period of time. **It is worth every penny!**

- Dr. Darlene Melk, Board Certified Pediatrician

Ashish, this is Russ Zwiener... **The weight of the world has been lifted! I have PASSED the 2018 ABP certifying exam. I improved my score by 42 points and passed by 35. Tears of joy are wonderful.** No Thank you could ever be sufficient for all the support and guidance over the past couple of years. Thank you again and please let me know if I could ever help with PBR in any way!!

Board Certified Pediatrician
VIP Bundle Member
"Deep Dive" call with Ashish
42-Point Increase
3 Prior failed attempts

The first time, I didn't finish... I landed a 166. The next year I joined PBR and went over the book 3 times. I should've taken off two weeks prior, but only managed one. I earned a 179. Heart breaking. But how could I give up when I only needed one point. So this year **I went over the book at least 5 more times. I did the ATL live test-taking strategies training and learned how to process through choosing the most correct answers.** I arranged to have at least 3 hrs of deep work everyday and did a chapter a day plus prep questions from that section. Two mos before the exam I did med study practice blocks of 84 questions timed to practice randomized subjects. **This time I got a 208...** The tears of relief...really I can't describe it as intensely as we felt it. So much time, work, money, defeat I had felt...finally redeemed. **The sacrifice my family made, finally we could leave purgatory and move on!** ... Thank you PBR.

Dr. Samantha
Board Certified Pediatrician
All Access Pass Member
Live Test-Taking Strategies & Deep Study Course Member
29-Point increase
2 Prior failed attempts

Ashish and Team. Today is the best day ever. I had to do many things to get here. **You gave me the tools, and my confidence back. The test taking strategies changed my approach to questions. It was clear, consistent and concise. I approached each question the same way. It took me 10 years to figure out how to take this test.** The personalized schedule kept me focused and on task. You helped me overcome my biggest challenge in my career. I passed with a 192. I am finally board certified after 10 years and I now have more options available to me. I can keep my family together. **I have conquered my biggest nemesis and it feels great!** You are awesome.

Dr. Cynthia Mondesir
Board Certified Pediatrician
All Access Pass Member
Live Test-Taking Strategies & Deep Study Course Member
"Deep Dive" call with Ashish
26-Point Increase
6 Prior attempts

> * All testimonials are by real people, and may not reflect the typical purchaser's experience, and are not intended to represent or guarantee that anyone will achieve the same or similar results.

The time that you spend learning <u>how</u> to use test-taking strategies to increase your scores will be the HIGHEST yield time of your board prep. The overall time investment is as little as 8-16 hours, but the skills you learn will be used on EVERY single question that you come across. Is there a single chapter in this book that can guarantee you the same benefit?

THE ANSWER IS "NO!"

① Signup for Your FREE Test-Taking Strategy Session Now

www.pediatricsboardreview.com/strategy

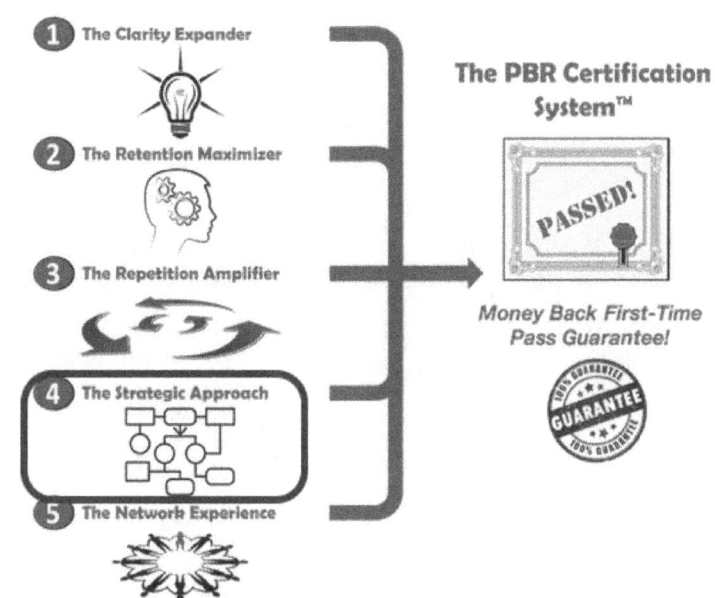

② Use the ONLINE Test-Taking Strategies Course

Go through the online course, do independent work, increase your skill, and reach a plateau.

www.pediatricsboardreview.com/strategy

③ Attend the LIVE Test-Taking Strategies & Deep Study Course

Come to the LIVE course, get mentored, maximize your test-taking strategy skills, BREAK THROUGH your plateau, and learn Deep Study techniques to maximize your "book time" too.

www.pediatricsboardreview.com/live-tts

DID YOU KNOW THAT I FAILED THE BOARDS?

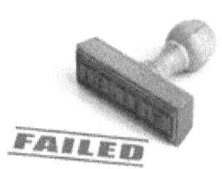

I took the ABP initial certification exam the year that I graduated from residency. **I used multiple study guides to prepare**. Because there was so much information in front of me (print and video), **I only got through everything once**.

I felt okay going into the exam. I thought, "I've been through the MCAT, three USMLE exams and an Internal Medicine board exam. I did fine in residency, and I studied really hard for two months. I'm *sure* I'll be fine."

Coming out of that exam room on test-day, I felt nauseous. I realized that I might have just failed my first medical board exam, ever! **I was upset with myself for getting so scattered with all of those different study materials**, but I was also annoyed because **I still couldn't think of a single resource that I could use as a primary study guide the next time around**.

I went home and made notes about **how I would study differently** if I had failed. What topics would I concentrate on? What topics just don't seem to be "testable"? What information is a waste of time to study?

When the results finally came, I failed. I estimate that I **failed by seven to nine questions. I made key strategy changes** based on my previous experience. I studied for hundreds of hours while still working a full-time job. I **focused on efficiency, solid mnemonics for memorization and I stopped trying to learn "all of pediatrics."**

You never feel "great" coming out of a board exam, but the second time around I felt like I had a fighting chance. **My score increased by 160 points on the old passing scale, and I estimated a pass by about 37–39 questions!** Pretty soon, I even received another kind of letter from the ABP. **The American Board of Pediatrics asked ME to write questions for the THEM!!!**

I was really just happy to pass. Failing **the first time had cost me extra time, money, and energy** that I would have preferred to spend with my loved ones.

Prior to creating the Pediatrics Board Review experience, I was ashamed that I had failed. Now, **I've taken a horrible experience, and I've created something that is helping residents and pediatrician across the country**. I've also realized that **failing the boards did not mean that I was a bad pediatrician**. Nor did passing by such a wide margin mean that I am a great pediatrician.

I'M JUST AN AVERAGE PERSON WHO DID EXTREMELY WELL ON THE EXAM… AND THEN TOOK MY NOTES AND SYSTEMS AND TURNED THEM INTO THE PBR. No matter who you are, I know that you can pass your exam too. That's why PBR comes with a **100% Money-Back First-Time Pass Guarantee**.

It's the easiest, most EFFICIENT, and only integrated board review *SYSTEM* to help you PASS the pediatric boards. So, rest assured that by joining the PBR family, you're already on the right track to success.

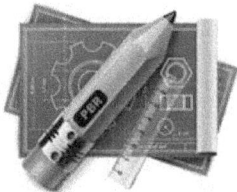

JUST FOLLOW THE EFFICIENCY BLUEPRINT!

THE PBR EFFICIENCY BLUEPRINT

The pediatric initial certification exam has **one of the highest failure rates of any medical board exam**. I URGE you to follow just a few of my simple but CRITICAL recommendations as you go through your board review experience. *ESPECIALLY #1*!

1. <u>**PLEASE STICK TO ONE PRIMARY STUDY GUIDE**</u> **- the PBR!** Spreading yourself too thin by reviewing multiple resources is the <u>***BIGGEST MISTAKE***</u> you can make. **I've gone through thousands of emails, interviews and surveys**. It's clear that this one, single recommendation that will increase your chances of board success more than anything else I can say.

   This is a **key similarity amongst pediatricians who failed** the boards but then went on to pass using the PBR system. So please **do not spend your time going through other books, video courses or expensive live board review courses. Go through the PBR books** (Core Study Guide + Q&A Book) **and the PBR companion products** (videos, MP3s, digital picture atlas, webinars) exclusively and give yourself a seamless, multimodal approach.

2. Approach your PBR material by first simply SEEING all of the PBR content in the Core Study Guide **and** Q&A Book. Spend about 60–90 seconds per page to simply SEE everything that you will need to learn so that you have an idea about the type of knowledge you'll need to acquire in order to pass this exam. **This should take you a full day. DO NOT spend time writing notes of any kind during this process.** Do NOT treat the Q&A Book like other questions. This is CORE content.

   During your first official read, leave no stone unturned. Crosscheck anything that confuses you. Create mnemonics, notes and drawings in the margins so that you understand EVERYTHING. Make sure that you will NEVER have to go outside of the PBR for additional knowledge or clarifications again. If you get stuck on a concept, reach **out to your peers in the PBR Community** (www.pbrlinks.com/**community**)! If you think you've found an error, notify us through our special error submission link (www.pediatricsboardreview.com/**error**). **This will help you maintain your PACE and promote EFFICIENCY!** When crosschecking, ONLY go outside of PBR briefly for possible errors or confusion. That's it! **Do NOT go down the black hole of GOOGLE!** If after 5 minutes you're still stuck, submit your question through the ASK THE EXPERT portal for that chapter and move on!

   Your second time should be MUCH faster if you are using <u>my highlighter system</u>. Do NOT let your curiosity of non-PBR topics distract you. As you break up your studying time with questions, you WILL want to look up new topics and crosscheck facts between the PBR and PREP®. DO NOT DO IT! It's a guaranteed waste of precious time that could be spent on the HIGHEST YIELD resources that you will have at your disposal to pass the board exam: PBR's.

   Your third, fourth and fifth times through the PBR content should strictly focus on adding more information into your long-term memory through <u>repetition</u>, through the use of mnemonics, and through the use of **MULTIMODAL studying**. Use audio, video, webinars, study buddy sessions, etc. Just use *something* to mix things up because it's been **proven to increase learning!** Use the audio course everywhere, and use the video course in a later "recapture" round (more on this in the members' area).

   Again, you must resist that urge to look up extraneous information and you must **focus on QUALITY study time**. Ensure that your reading is focused on LEARNING and REMEMBERING the concepts. Do not simply read for the sake of reading, and do not study when you're exhausted or irritable.

   Your primary goal is to <u>pass the exam</u>. As long as you KNOW everything from the Core Study Guide + Q&A Book, **you will have enough information in your brain to easily pass as long as you also have good test-taking strategy. However, if you try to learn "all of pediatrics"** you will get overwhelmed and probably **fail the exam**. Map out the right number of hours based on your risk profile (more on this coming up) and hold yourself accountable.

3. **Use PBR's Q&A book as additional, new CORE material. Also use it to get familiar with very high-yield topics and questions**. The format is short and to the point without too much extra information. The questions will help you understand what types of key findings you need to identify on your practice questions and on your exam. Please remember that **the Q&A book is considered CORE CONTENT**. You need to KNOW IT COLD! Do NOT treat the PBR questions like PREP® questions.

4. **Go through at least 1000 practice questions.** Don't go through them all at once (much more on this in the schedule outlines below). As you go through the questions, **work on your timing**. If you can average about 1 minute and 15 seconds per question, you will be fine for the boards. Do not try to understand why every single incorrect answer is wrong. **Just focus on the correct answer, and if your answer is wrong, figure out WHY it's wrong.** Skip explanations about all of the other answer choices.

    When evaluating WHY you answered a question wrong, figure out if it was because of a **CONTENT problem** or if it was due to a **TECHNIQUE problem**. Even if you "think" you're sure, trust me, it could still be a TECHNIQUE problem, and you must get help – www.pediatricsboardreview.com/strategies.

    Did you answer a question incorrectly because of a CONTENT issue? Meaning, you had a knowledge deficiency? If so, was the content in the PBR? If the answer is "yes" then you MUST know that information. If the answer is "no" then do NOT worry about it! Do NOT start looking at Nelson's, Harriet Lane, Google, UpToDate, etc. **It's a black hole that you must avoid** because it will only overwhelm you, and it will keep you from the two main goals of **knowing the PBR CONTENT COLD** and **PRACTICING tons of questions** to master your test-taking technique!

    Remember, the AAP writes PREP®, the ABP writes the boards. Going through **three to four years of PREP®** is great, but keep in mind that the resource is great for **CME**. Any single year of PREP® questions is *not* designed to be a stand-alone study guide for the ABP exam. The questions are EXCELLENT for practicing and mastering your test-taking technique, but your highest-yield information will come from the PBR study guides and systems. If you need MORE practice questions, you can get discounted practice questions by visiting www.pediatricsboardreview.com/tools.

    Did you answer a question incorrectly because of a TECHNIQUE issue? Did you add extra information and assumptions to the question or the answers that led you to the wrong answer? Did you spend too much time on a question even though it was clear that you didn't have the knowledge to answer it? **Did the question-writer trick you with a distractor?** Did the question writer trick you with an English question instead of a clinical question? Did you get anxious or nervous under a timed mock exam? **Did you often get stuck between seemingly similar answer choices?** Are you still confused about why the answer you chose is wrong?

    Make notes about the kinds of issues you're having and try to figure out solution and strategies to avoid similar pitfalls in the future. If you notice that TECHNIQUES-BASED PROBLEMS creeping in over and over again, or you don't know what I mean by "technique," you need to **seek out help through the PBR Test-Taking Strategies & Coaching course at** www.pediatricsboardreview.com/strategies.

5. **EXTREMELY Important Test Day Tips**: PLAN to be successful. You will find two links below. The first breaks down the number of questions, time per block, etc. for your exam. The second is **a list of excellent PBR articles**.

    www.pediatricsboardreview.com/examday

    www.pediatricsboardreview.com/category/test-day-tips

STUDY SCHEDULE: Resident? First-Time? Failed? MOC? MOCA? WE'VE GOT YOU TAKEN CARE OF!

We have a TON of guidance on how you can schedule your study time. Since PBR is of benefit to pediatricians at all different levels, I've tailored my recommendations accordingly below.

EVERYONE MUST recognize the **difference between clinical practice and what the ABP would want you to do on the exam**. The exam is filled with answer choices that sound like they would be great options in practice, but unless you know what "the book" says, you will have to simply roll the dice.

For anyone taking the **Initial Certification exam**, recognize that the pass rates are DRAMATICALLY LOWER than the USMLE Step Exams. **In 2023, the first-time pass rate for US and Canadian medical students taking the USMLE Step 1 was approximately 92% while the pass rate for the ABP initial certification exam was only 82%!** Our members' pass rate for first-time test takers of the ABP exams is estimated to be > 98%! So, stay focused on PBR!

ARE YOU A RESIDENT? Simply familiarizing yourself with everything in the PBR content before you graduate will dramatically increase your chances of passing the boards.

While on subspecialty rotations, READ and KNOW the associated PBR chapter. While on general inpatient or outpatient rotations, focus on the rest of the book, and take just 15 minutes per day to read the QUICK and high-yield topics about your patients. Pace yourself so that you can get through the material at least once per year. That's it! If you do that, your in-training scores will skyrocket, and you will DESTROY the boards.

ARE YOU TAKING THE INITIAL EXAM FOR THE FIRST TIME? If your PBR risk assessment shows that you are a low-risk test-taker, that likely means you're a first-time test-taker, you're taking the exam immediately after residency, and you have **never come close to failing** a medical board exam (above average board scores). Visit the following PBR article for a detailed study schedule:

www.pediatricsboardreview.com/**Schedule**

HAVE YOU EVER FAILED A MEDICAL BOARD EXAM (OR COME CLOSE)? If your PBR risk assessment shows that you are at moderate or high risk of failing the boards, you were likely categorized as being "at risk" of failing based on your in-training exam scores, you may have failed a medical board exam (ANY medical board exam) previously, or you generally score **below the national average on your board exams**. Visit the following PBR article for detailed instructions on how you can avoid failing your pediatric boards:

www.pediatricsboardreview.com/**Schedule-Failed**

ARE YOU STUDYING FOR MOCA-PEDS? For the "at home," MOCA-Peds questions, the plan is simple. Use the **MOCA-PBR Study Guide & Test Companion**. Go through our concise summaries of the most current year's Learning Objectives in detail one time. It may only take you a single day! Since MOCA-PBR is setup to be an efficient test companion to help you with your open book exam, keep it open as you do your MOCA-Peds questions. Review your MOCA-PBR study guide once per quarter. That's it!

www.pediatricsboardreview.com/**MOCA**

ARE YOU STUDYING FOR THE MOC? If you are taking the pediatric recertification exam, then your goal should be to get through the PBR materials at least twice and to do at least 550 practice questions. Did you know that you may have access to **200 FREE ABP questions**. Go through them!

www.pediatricsboardreview.com/**MOC**

TIPS FOR YOUR STUDYING & TEST-TAKING EFFICIENCY

1. DO NOT treat this Q&A book as any other question bank. Study it as many times as you plan on studying your PBR Core Study Guide. Treat it as "core content". Use a variety of other question banks as disposable questions that are used to help you practice your **test-taking strategy**.

2. Study as though you are going to be a general pediatrician, or a pediatrician practicing in an ER setting. You are not expected to know the deeper management of complicated topics that would require a specialist's involvement. You are expected to know the initial management.

3. Know normal lab values for common labs (including Hgb, Hct, Plt, WBC, albumin, chemistry panel, etc.).

4. Do not memorize reference range values for uncommon labs.

5. Know how to interpret the results of an ABG in the setting of acid-base disorders.

6. Do not try to go through an entire image atlas.

7. Becoming familiar with high-yield images is recommended but know that you can pass the boards without having a strong handle on the images. For some of you, your time is likely going to be better spent going through the core study guide over and over again and just ignoring the images. If you have time, use PBR's online image links to quickly and efficiently become familiar with hundreds of high-yield images. Be mentally prepared to see a handful of questions in which you are asked to identify a disease process or disease association on the basis of only a single image.

8. Do NOT worry about memorizing epidemiologic percentages. Just have a feel for what diseases are more common than others.

9. Focus, focus and focus some more on using PBR as your primary study resource so that you don't get too distracted by other materials. After you've gone through PBR five times, feel free to go through as many other resources as you want.

10. **Use MULTIPLE question banks to practice your test-taking strategy. Don't try to finish all of the questions for a given Q bank. It's more important that you learn test-taking strategies and then start to apply them to different question banks. Use the questions as a tool to hone your skill rather than a source of more content!**

11. For EXTREMELY **Important Test Day Tips visit**

    www.pediatricsboardreview.com/category/test-day-tips

FORMAT OF THE PBR Q&A SECTIONS

Ready for some questions? This book contains 50 extremely high-yield questions. You will be presented with sections of questions followed by sections of answers. Each section contains approximately 5-10 questions/answers.

NOTE: Several questions contain information not covered in the core study guide. Please be sure to go over this material several times as many times as you are expected to go over the PBR core study guide (FIVE)!

PRODUCT REGISTRATION

As mentioned on the PBR site, our first-time pass guarantee applies to anyone taking an ABP initial or recertification exam for the first time. "Money Back" requests may be made within 30 days of the score release date. The original PBR purchase must have been made at least 45 days prior to the exam. Submission of the product registration form is required for the money back pass guarantee and the form must be submitted within 90 days of your purchase and before you take the exam. For complete details, please visit:

www.pediatricsboardreview.com/guarantee

Visit the following link to register your product(s):

www.pediatricsboardreview.com/register

If you made an official purchase that was initiated through the PBR website but resulted in your purchase being processed through Lulu.com, Amazon.com, or another authorized distributor of PBR resources, please contact us through www.pediatricsboardreview.com/contact so that you can send us a copy of your receipt.

QUESTIONS

1. A premature baby needs:
   a. More sodium than a full-term neonate. Sodium supplementation should be started immediately.
   b. More sodium than a full-term neonate. Sodium supplementation can be started after 24 hours.
   c. Less sodium than a full-term baby.
   d. The same amount of sodium as a full-term baby.

2. A preemie is born at 33 weeks in a taxi. In the ER, the baby is noted to have a temperature of 35 degrees Celsius. The child should be placed:
   a. In a bassinette.
   b. In an incubator at 40 degrees Celsius.
   c. Under a radiant warmer at maximum temperature.
   d. Under a radiant warmer at preferred skin temperature.

3. An LGA baby is noted to have a firm, freely mobile, erythematous and nodular mass with distinct borders at the upper cheek on DOL 13. This is likely:
   a. Fat necrosis of the newborn.
   b. A lipoma
   c. A sarcoma
   d. Related to child abuse.

4. Which abnormality is common in the recipient of a packed red blood cell (PRBC) transfusion and also in the recipient twin of a twin-to-twin transfusion?
   a. Hyponatremia
   b. Hypokalemia
   c. Hypocalcemia
   d. Hypophosphatemia

5. A child is born by a normal vaginal delivery. About 8 hours later he is noted to be tachypneic and pale. Labs show that he is anemic. The RBC morphology is normal under microscopy. What is the likely etiology of these finding?
   a. Chronic intrauterine blood loss.
   b. Acute blood loss at birth.
   c. Congenital heart disease.
   d. Congenital syphilis

ANSWERS

1. The answer is B, *"More sodium than a full-term neonate. Sodium supplementation can be started after 24 hours."* Premature babies have an increased fractional excretion of sodium (FENa) due to poor sodium reabsorption. The GFR and the sodium reabsorption improves with age. Sodium supplementation is not needed in the first 24 hours. Assume this is due to the initial water losses.
    a. PEARL: In VLBW babies, water losses can **exceed** sodium losses. This can actually result in **hypernatremia** if enough free water is not provided.

2. The answer is D, *"Under a radiant warmer at preferred skin temperature."* The child is too hypothermic to put in a bassinette. Placing a preemie in an incubator at 40 degrees Celsius, or under a radiant warmer at the maximum temperature would overheat the child. Also, the typical set point for an incubator is 36.5 – 37.4 degrees.
    a. PEARLS: Incubator temperatures can be difficult to control, so it's good to have the baby under a warmer while work is being done in the ER. Otherwise, a great deal of warmth is lost when the door is opened. In general, radiant warmers tend to be associated with less morbidity. Check temperature frequently. Move the baby to a **pre-warmed** incubator once the door will not be opened frequently.

3. The answer is A, *"Fat necrosis of the newborn"* is a condition of unknown etiology. LGA status is a definite risk factor. Also, any child with a perinatal event (meconium aspiration, trauma, asphyxia, etc.) is at increased risk. It's self-limited, but can be complicated by **hypercalcemia that can be life-threatening**. Look for a nodular lesion at the **cheeks, thighs, buttocks or arms**. No treatment, but do check electrolytes including calcium.
    a. PEARL: Cold exposure is another risk factor and the same findings could be referred to as a cold induced panniculitis. Look for a child with a pacifier filled with cold water. S/he will be afebrile.

4. The answer is C, *"Hypocalcemia"* is a common transfusion related reaction, both in twin-to-twin transfusions and in regular PRBC transfusions. **Hyper**kalemia and thrombocytopenia are also common in regular PRBC transfusions. Consider using the mnemonics below to remember these findings.
    a. MNEMONICS: A usual PRBC transfusion is 10-20 cc/kg. Think of it as a giving a "bolus" of PRBCs (a "bolus" of IVF is 20 cc/kg). Regarding complications, think of calcium precipitating out as the 2 different bloods mix (actually it's a citrate toxicity). For the hyperkalemia, imagine RBCs hemolyzing as they get sheared through the IV. For thrombocytopenia, just assume it's a hemodilutional effect!

5. The answer is B, *"Acute blood loss at birth."* Only A and B should have been on your radar. The normal RBC morphology should have tipped you off to the acuity of the problem. For a chronic anemia, you would also expect a fairly stable patient.

QUESTIONS

6. A 40-year-old pregnant woman has a previous child with Down syndrome. She is now 15 weeks pregnant. What is the most appropriate recommendation for her?

    a. No special testing
    b. Maternal triple screen including HCG subunit
    c. Amniocentesis
    d. Chorionic villus sampling

7. A pregnant woman is being evaluated at 32 weeks gestation. The fetus is noted to have frequent premature heart beat on the monitor. The baby is having anywhere from 6-10 premature beats per minute. They are usually individual, but up to 3 have been noted in succession. The woman drinks 1 cup of coffee per day. What's the next step?

    a. No workup is indicated
    b. Obtain a fetal echocardiogram
    c. Recommend cessation of all caffeine intake and recheck in one week
    d. Do a urine toxicology screen on the mother

8. A woman is in labor with a full-term child. She has one other child and states that he had a "Strep problem" after being born and needed IV antibiotics. She had a UTI 4 weeks ago and was given antibiotics. She had a GBS screen 3 weeks ago, which was negative. What is the next best step?

    a. Send a stat GBS screen
    b. Do nothing because GBS prophylaxis is not indicated.
    c. Give GBS prophylaxis immediately.
    d. Let her deliver by vaginal delivery and then monitor the child for 48 hours before allowing discharge.

9. A child has a history of Tetralogy of Fallot is noted to have a Tet spell. He looks fairly cyanotic on exam. All of the following medications can be given during an acute Tet spell EXCEPT:

    a. Morphine
    b. Phenobarbital
    c. Phenylephrine
    d. Metoprolol

10. A neonate develops respiratory distress and pulse oximetry shows declining saturations. A chest X-ray is shown. You note diffuse, fluffy interstitial infiltrates. Which medication do you give next?

    a. Furosemide
    b. Prostaglandin

11. A neonate develops declining oxygen saturations on DOL 1. Capillary refill is slow and central cyanosis is noted. A chest X-ray is shown. You note clear lung fields. Which medication do you give next?

    a. Furosemide

    b. Prostacyclin

12. You are shown an image of a newborn. He has what looks like a thin, transparent film on his body. Eyelashes are missing and eyelids seem inverted (IMAGE: www.pbrlinks.com/QA12). What is the diagnosis?

    a. Lamellar ichthyosis

    b. Harlequin ichthyosis

    c. Lichen striatus

    d. Ichthyosis vulgaris

13. A 5-month-old male presents for a well-child visit. The child's brother had developmental dysplasia of the hip. The patient has no extra folds and both the Barlow and Ortolani maneuvers are negative. The mother asks if this child needs to have any special tests done. What is the next best step in management?

    a. Ultrasound of the hips.

    b. Hip X-rays.

    c. Reassure the mother that this child has a normal exam, but recommend follow up with an orthopedist for further evaluation and risk stratification.

    d. Inform the mother that her son has a normal exam and he does not need any imaging studies.

14. A child is born with choanal atresia, a cleft palate and syndactyly in his upper and lower extremities. He's discharged from the hospital and is noted to have early suture closure over the coming months. Two images are shown (www.pbrlinks.com/QA14A & www.pbrlinks.com/QA14B). What disorder does the child have?

    a. Smith-Lemli-Opitz

    b. Crouzon Syndrome

    c. Pierre-Robin Syndrome

    d. Apert Syndrome

15. A baby girl is born at home in a tub. She was given a dose of oral vitamin K and is being breastfed. On DOL 3, the child starts to have sudden bleeding noted in her diaper. What's the most likely diagnosis?

    a. Factor VIII Deficiency

    b. Factor IX Deficiency

    c. Factor X Deficiency

    d. Hemorrhagic Disease of the Newborn

ANSWERS

6. The answer is C, "*amniocentesis*" She is considered high risk for having another Trisomy 21 child (Down Syndrome = Trisomy 21) for multiple reasons (age + history of prior DS baby). It's a good idea to be familiar with date cutoffs for the different trimesters (2nd begins with the 13th week, 3rd begins with the 29th week), and the different tests that can be offered for DS screening in first and second trimesters.

    a. AMNIOCENTESIS: Generally considered a 2nd trimester option. This is usually offered as a screen at 15-18 weeks for women over the age of 35. It can be offered earlier, at 12 weeks, in certain circumstances. For high-risk women, this is the preferred test since it is more sensitive and specific than serum testing. It is also less risky than CVS.

    b. CHORIONIC VILLUS TESTING: Generally considered a 2nd trimester option, but this can also be done as early as 12 weeks. It is more definitive but carries more risks, including an increased chance of miscarriage, when compared to amniocentesis.

    c. MATERNAL SERUM TRIPLE OR QUADRUPLE SCREEN: Considered to be 2nd trimester options. These include obtaining 3-4 of the serum markers noted below.

        - AFP: Low is bad.
        - Unconjugated estriol: Low is bad
        - Beta HCG subunit: High is bad
        - Inhibin (for the quadruple screen): High is bad

    d. FIRST TRIMESTER OPTION: The usual first trimester option includes using a combination of ultrasound and serum HCG subunit testing late in the first trimester. The ultrasound is done to look for **nuchal translucency.** If that is found along with an elevated beta HCG, there's a high chance of the baby having Down Syndrome.

7. The answer is B, "*Obtain a fetal echocardiogram.*" Premature beats in a fetus are not normal and warrant a workup for congenital heart disease. A fetal echocardiogram should be done as soon as possible. If congenital heart disease exists, then precautions will need to be in place at the time of delivery.

    a. PEARL: In an older child, 3-4 PVCs per minute are generally allowed. Six or more should be investigated further. Start with checking electrolytes and obtaining a 12-lead EKG.

8. The answer is C, "*Give GBS prophylaxis immediately.*" GBS prophylaxis **is** indicated because of possible invasive GBS disease in a **previous** infant. Here is your GBS screening & prophylaxis made easy!

    a. RECTOVAGINAL GROUP B BETA HEMOLYTIC STREPTOCOCCUS (GBS) SCREENING CULTURES: These are obtained at **36 to 37 6/7 weeks gestation**.

    b. INTRAPARTUM ANTIBIOTIC PROPHYLAXIS (IAP): Intrapartum Antibiotic Prophylaxis (IAP) refers to antibiotics given to mom when she presents for delivery. If indicated, give IV penicillin, ampicillin or cefazolin at least 4 hours prior to delivery. The latest guidelines from the CDC may be viewed for some "light reading" by visiting www.pbrlinks.com/gbsprophylaxis.

    c. TO GIVE OR NOT TO GIVE INTRAPARTUM ANTIBIOTIC PROPHYLAXIS? IAP is indicated for any of the following scenarios:

        i. Invasive GBS disease was present in a **previous** infant
        ii. Positive GBS was noted in the URINE at ANYTIME during **THIS** pregnancy (regardless of treatment and subsequent cultures)

- iii. Positive rectovaginal GBS screening culture noted 36 to 37 6/7 weeks in **THIS** pregnancy
- iv. Unknown GBS status PLUS any of these:
    1. < 37 weeks gestation
    2. ROM > 18 hours
    3. Intrapartum fever of > 100.4 F
    4. Positive intrapartum NAAT testing
  d. IAP is considered "adequate" when penicillin, ampicillin or cefazolin is administered ≥ 4 hours prior to delivery.
  e. IAP is NOT indicated for GBS positivity in previous pregnancies or for c-sections done with intact membranes.

9. The answer is B, "*Phenobarbital*" Tet spells can result in cyanosis or even syncope and collapse as there is insufficient blood return to the pulmonary vasculature due to increased right to left shunting. First, a child should squat in order to increase blood return to the pulmonary artery. In younger children, the knees should be brought up to their chests. If that doesn't work and the child ends up in the ER, **morphine** is usually the first-line agent. If that doesn't work, then IV beta blockers or vasopressors may be used. IVF may also be given. Neither calcium channel blockers nor phenobarbital have a role in Tet spells.

10. The answer is A, "*Furosemide*" See next answer for explanation.

11. The answer is B, "*Prostacyclin*" Treatment of cardiac disease in a neonate or infant can be challenging. These two questions are meant to help you focus on a few key findings to look for, including age, presence of cyanosis, and chest X-ray findings. Hopefully, you will be given enough information to mentally diagnose a condition and provide management accordingly. If not, use the following rules to help guide you:

    a. CYANOSIS IN A NEONATE < 7 DAYS OLD: Give PROSTAGLANDIN or PROSTACYCLIN. For your purposes, the two are synonymous. The quickest way to get blood to the lungs for oxygenation is by maintaining the ductus arteriosus. The high pressure from the aorta will force blood into the pulmonary artery.

    b. RESPIRATORY DISTRESS OR CYANOSIS WITH A CLEAR CHEST X-RAY: Give PROSTAGLANDIN or PROSTACYCLIN. A **CLEAR** chest X-ray (or one that looks "too clear"), suggests there is not enough blood getting to the lungs. Giving PGE will change that through the mechanism discussed above.

    c. EVIDENCE OF PULMONARY EDEMA: Hopefully this will be seen in a patient after DOL 1. If so, give FUROSEMIDE or another diuretic. Fluffy infiltrates mean there is pulmonary congestion/edema. This can happen due to a septal defect, a PDA or other reasons. The point is, if a child is in a fluid overloaded situation, then help remove fluid with a diuretic.

    d. NOTE: Please note that the above rules are meant to guide you when you're not sure of a diagnosis, but have been able to recognize at least a few key findings.

12. The answer is A, "*Lamellar ichthyosis*" This is a classic description and image of lamellar ichthyosis. Of the choices, it should only be confused with harlequin ichthyosis, which also presents at birth, but is more severe. Harlequin ichthyosis is described as presenting with a hard and horny ("armor-like") covering. Prognosis is comparatively poor (www.pbrlinks.com/HARLEQUIN1).

13. The answer is B, "*Hip X-rays*". DEVELOPMENTAL DYSPLASIA OF THE HIP – Infants with developmental dysplasia of the hip (DDH) may be noted to have a leg-length discrepancy, extra creases

at the thigh, "clunks" or "clicks" on exam. A majority of newborn "clunks" resolve by 2 weeks of age. So do NOT obtain any imaging at the time of birth. ALL patients with an unequivocal Barlow or Ortolani maneuver (meaning there's no question in your mind on exam), limited hip abduction, or asymmetric hip abduction after 1 month should be referred to an orthopedist for evaluation. For children **6 weeks-4 months of age, ultrasound** should be used. After **4 months of age, hip x-rays should be used**. Treatment of DDH requires a Pavlik harness.

PEARL: Consider imaging before 6 months of age for any male or female infant with normal findings on physical exam, but any of the following risk factors.

- Breech presentation in the third trimester
- Positive family history
- History of previous clinical instability
- Parental concern
- History of improper swaddling
- Suspicious or inconclusive physical exam

PEARL: Ultrasound can be used from 6 weeks to 6 months and radiographs are recommended > 4 months. Radiographs are preferred after 4 months due to the lower rate of false positives compared to ultrasound. NEVER image before 2 weeks of age. For a child with no clinical signs of DDH on exam but with a NEED for evaluation based on high risk factors, you can ultrasound at 6 weeks or obtain radiographs at 4 months of age. When it comes to the Barlow and Ortolani signs, if EITHER of them is positive, send for imaging (after 2 weeks of age)! ALL children should be "screened" periodically at the well-child visits by EXAM! Meaning, if you're asked if you should "screen" a child for DDH at the 2-month visit, the answer is always going to be YES. Lastly, if you encounter an asymptomatic child that was supposed to get imaging (e.g., breech, family history) but never did, and the patient is now 5 or 6 months old, GET IMAGING even if the exam is normal!

IMAGE: www.pbrlinks.com/DDH1

IMAGE: www.pbrlinks.com/DDH2

14. The answer is D, "*Apert Syndrome*" Patients with Apert syndrome can have the 4 features mentioned (bilateral syndactyly, craniosynostosis, cleft palate and choanal atresia). Inheritance is autosomal dominant. Most cases are from sporadic mutations because of poor reproductive fitness. Crouzon has craniosynostosis, but NOT syndactyly. Smith-Lemli-Opitz syndrome has 2-3 syndactyly. Pierre-Robin syndrome can have syndactyly, but the other symptoms do not fit.

    a. PEARL: Craniosynostosis (early suture closure) + BILATERAL syndactyly = PICK APERT on the exam! Unilateral syndactyly is probably something else.
    b. MNEMONIC: "APERT" is French and pronounced "A PEAR." Imagine A PEAR-shaped head! Imagine the cranium being small because of early suture closure. Imagining A PEAR-shaped APERT head could KEEP you from guessing ALPERS or ALPORT on the exam.

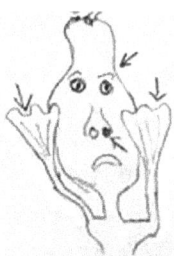

15. The answer is D, "*Hemorrhagic Disease of the Newborn*" For Hemophilia A, Hemophilia B and Factor X deficiency, look for bleeding due to minor trauma. Factor X deficiency can have mild spontaneous

bleeding. Vitamin K deficiency (Phytonadione deficiency) can result in HEMORRHAGIC DISEASE OF THE NEWBORN due to a coagulopathy. Vitamin K is needed for use with coagulation factors 2, 7, 9, and 10. This is especially a concern in babies because there is a lack of normal gut flora needed to make the Vitamin K. Deficiency is also more common in breastfed babies that did not receive Vitamin K at birth (watch out for a home birth). Look for a bleeding circumcision site or umbilical cord site.

    a. PEARL: Oral Vitamin K at birth does NOT prevent HEMORRHAGIC DISEASE OF THE NEWBORN.

    b. Early Vitamin K deficiency usually occurs within the first week of life.

    c. Late Vitamin K deficiency can occur any time between two weeks and three months! Look for a breastfed baby on antibiotics who has diarrhea (decreased gut flora to make Vitamin K due to antibiotic use, and decreased absorption due to diarrhea).

    d. TREATMENT: For bleeding patients, give Vitamin K + FFP (fresh frozen plasma contains plenty of functional Vitamin K dependent coagulation factors).

QUESTIONS

16. A child is noted to have jaundice on DOL 1 at approximately 20 hours birth. There is a family history of physiologic jaundice. The child is being breastfed by his Rh+ mother. What is the most likely diagnosis?

    a. Physiologic jaundice
    b. Rhesus disease
    c. Breast milk jaundice
    d. TORCH Infection

17. On DOL 3, a child is noted to have jaundice and a total bilirubin of 10. The baby is formula feeding well. The mother received appropriate prenatal care and workup for Rh disease and ABO incompatibility is negative. What is the next best step in management?

    a. Discharge with follow-up in 48 hours
    b. Start phototherapy
    c. Start IV fluids
    d. Prepare for plasma exchange

18. A newborn is noted to have jaundice at 48 hours of life. Labs show a predominantly indirect hyperbilirubinemia with a total bilirubin level is 10. The child is formula feeding well. The child was born at 37 weeks gestation, has a brother who required phototherapy, and has a small cephalohematoma. What's the next step in management?

    a. No intervention is needed
    b. Recheck bilirubin in 8 hours
    c. Start phototherapy
    d. Obtain a stat right upper quadrant ultrasound

19. A crying 3-year old child is shown with macroglossia (macroglossia image: www.pbrlinks.com/QA19A). The child seems to have microcephaly and has a history of an umbilical hernia. What's the most likely diagnosis?

    a. Hypothyroidism
    b. Down Syndrome
    c. Pierre-Robin Syndrome
    d. Beckwith-Wiedemann Syndrome

20. A newborn baby boy is noted to have small hands and hypotonia. Magnesium sulfate tocolysis was given to the mother. The child's hypotonia is most likely due to:
    a. Magnesium sulfate
    b. Hypothyroidism
    c. Prader-Willi Syndrome
    d. Achondroplasia

21. A newborn baby boy is noted to have a case of glandular hypospadias, in which the opening is displaced, but still on the glans. The family requests that the boy be circumcised. The next best step in management is to:
    a. Move forward with a circumcision and then refer the patient to urology for a future correction.
    b. Move forward with a circumcision. The child does qualify for surgical correction.
    c. Refer to urology for surgical correction.
    d. Obtain a karyotype.

22. A male newborn had oligohydramnios noted on prenatal ultrasound. You examine the child a few hours after the delivery and are unable to palpate testicles in the scrotum. The child has not produced urine yet, and you note a very soft abdomen with a midline abdominal mass. Which of the following is the most likely diagnosis?
    a. Congenital adrenal hyperplasia
    b. Prune Belly Syndrome
    c. Wilms Tumor
    d. Kallmann Syndrome

23. A newborn is noted to have a distended abdomen and bilious emesis. It has been 24 hours and meconium has not been passed. A contrast study (similar to the one here www.pbrlinks.com/QA23A) shows contrast throughout the colon. Which of the following is the most likely diagnosis?
    a. Malrotation
    b. Duodenal atresia
    c. Microcolon
    d. Intussusception

24. An 18-year-old teen gets pregnant after her first sexual encounter. She has an uncomplicated pregnancy and received adequate prenatal care. Soon after birth, the newborn is found to be jaundiced. The child is found to have a total bilirubin of 13. A blood smear shows spherocytes. The mother's blood type is O, Rh-. The newborn's blood type is A, Rh+. What is the most likely cause of the hyperbilirubinemia?
    a. ABO incompatibility
    b. Rhesus disease
    c. Hereditary spherocytosis
    d. Biliary atresia

ANSWERS

16. The answer is D, "*TORCH Infection*" Any time you see jaundice within the first 24 hours of life, that is BAD. Physiologic jaundice is a diagnosis of exclusion and usually occurs on DOL 3 or 2 at the earliest. Rh disease occurs in Rh- mothers. Breast **milk** jaundice usually occurs at about 1 week, though it can present earlier (this is not the same thing as breastfeeding jaundice). That only leaves the TORCH infections. Please see #17 for more.

17. The answer is A, "*Discharge with follow-up in 48 hours*" This child has PHYSIOLOGIC JAUNDICE. Physiologic jaundice is a **diagnosis of exclusion**. Look for a healthy infant with jaundice on DOL 2 through 5 with no pathologic explanation. Make sure somewhat of a workup has been done.

    a. PEARLS: KNOW AS MUCH AS YOU CAN ABOUT JAUNDICE AND HYPERBILIRUBINEMIA. The placenta clears unconjugated bilirubin in utero. The enzyme needed to conjugate the unconjugated (indirect) bilirubin to conjugated (direct) bilirubin can take some time to mature after birth. Jaundice within the first 24 hours should be investigated further with a direct and indirect bilirubin level. **DIRECT hyperbilirubinemia** in the newborn is ALWAYS BAD, and means there is serious pathology (likely a biliary obstruction). Any direct bilirubinemia > 1 is abnormal. **DO NOT** order phototherapy in a baby with direct hyperbilirubinemia because it can cause "bronze baby syndrome." **Indirect hyperbilirubinemia** could mean one of many disorders, including hemolysis (consider G6PD if male), prematurity, hypothyroidism, a genetic defect/enzyme deficiency (galactosemia, Crigler Najjar), sepsis or certain congenital TORCH infection. In an older child with a mild indirect bilirubinemia during an illness, it could also mean Gilbert syndrome (very benign).

    b. PEARL: Use of alcohol, heroin, phenobarbital, phenytoin and tobacco are all associated with a DECREASED risk of hyperbilirubinemia.

18. The answer is A "*No intervention is needed*" The child is at high risk, but does not need phototherapy and may be discharged.

    a. RISK FACTORS FOR DEVELOPING HYPERBILIRUBINEMIA: G6PD deficiency, asphyxia, temperature instability, sepsis, acidosis, albumin < 3, ABO incompatibility, Rh disease, sibling with history of phototherapy, bruising, cephalohematoma and exclusive breastfeeding that is not going well. SO ALMOST ANYTHING IS A RISK FACTOR. Focus instead on identifying neonates that are at high and medium risk of developing hyperbilirubinemia, as well as memorizing the bilirubin levels at which phototherapy should be initiated.

    b. **HIGHEST RISK BABIES:** 35 – 37 + 6/7 weeks WITH risk factors

    c. MEDIUM RISK BABIES: 35 – 37 + 6/7 weeks WITHOUT risk factors. OR, > 38 weeks WITH risk factors.

    d. LOW RISK BABIES: >38 weeks and well

    e. START PHOTOTHERAPY ON **HIGH** RISK NEONATES IF:

        - **TOTAL** bilirubin >**8 at 24 hours**
        - **TOTAL** bilirubin >**11 at 48 hours**
        - **TOTAL** bilirubin >**13 at 72 hours**

    f. SHORTCUTS FOR WHEN TO START PHOTOTHERAPY IN MEDIUM & LOW RISK NEONATES:

        - MEDIUM risk: The bilirubin threshold increases by 2 (so approximately 10, 13, and 15).

- LOW risk: The bilirubin threshold increases by 4 (so approximately 12, 15 and 18).
  g. PEARL: NONE OF THE ABOVE-MENTIONED RISK FACTORS AND BILIRUBIN THRESHOLDS APPLY TO PREMATURE NEONATES < 35 WEEKS.

19. The answer is D, "Beckwith-Wiedemann Syndrome" BECKWITH-WIEDEMANN: Look for MACROglossia, MICROcephaly, MACROsomia (large body), midline abdominal wall defects and evidence of **hemihypertrophy (AKA hemihyperplasia)**. The midline defect may be an omphalocele (bowel through the umbilicus) or umbilical hernia. Babies will often have neonatal hypoglycemia. Children are at increased risk for malignancies, especially Wilms Tumor. Look for a picture of a patient with a big body, big tongue and some type of overgrowth symptom (unilateral overgrowth of a leg, face, arm, etc.).
    a. PEARL: It's the most common overgrowth syndrome in infancy and it would be VERY, VERY worthwhile to learn about it.
    b. IMAGE: www.pbrlinks.com/QA19B
    c. IMAGE: www.pbrlinks.com/QA19C
    d. MNEMONIC: Replace the "W's" with "V's". Rename it BeckVvith-VvIDE mouth. The different sized V's are to remind you of the hemihypertrophy (often seen on the ABP exam). The "Vvide mouth" is needed to accommodate the large tongue in this very small head!

20. The answer is C, "*Prader-Willi Syndrome*" The rest can cause hypotonia, and achondroplasia can be associated with "trident-like" fingers, but not small hands.
    a. **Prader-Willi syndrome** (AKA Prader Willi syndrome) patients can have hypotonia (floppy baby), mild retardation, almond-shaped eyes (often with mild strabismus), small hands, a HUGE appetite, obesity, and small testicles/penis in boys.
        i. * **PEARLS:** Like Angelman's, it can be found in BOYS or GIRLS. This mechanism of this disorder is the mirror image of that of Angelman's. It occurs due to the absence or dysfunction of the PATERNAL copy of a gene in the same region of chromosome 15 as in Angelman syndrome. It also occurs when two maternal copies of chromosome 15 were received and no paternal copies (maternal disomy), and also when a mutation of the paternal gene makes it behave like the MATERNAL gene (called maternal imprinting). Symptoms are much milder in females. The gene location is probably not important for the test, but the fact that it is KNOWN (15q11-13) means that this disorder can be diagnosed by FISH.
        ii. **IMAGE**: www.pbrlinks.com/PRADERWILLI1
        iii. **IMAGE**: www.pbrlinks.com/PRADERWILLI2
        iv. **MNEMONIC:** Imagine a FAT Will Smith with TINY HANDS shoving tons of ALMONDS in his mouth. He's wearing a t-shirt that says, "MOMMY'S LITTLE FATTY."
            1. **KEY:** ALMONDS represent the shape of the eyes, and the t-shirt represents maternal imprinting.
        v. **MNEMONIC:** Sorry, this is a good mnemonic but not politically correct. Imagine a HUGE, OBESE, and DUMB FISH/WHALE named FREE WILLY with such a SMALL PENIS that you can hardly see it. It's so DUMB that it tried to jump over a dock, but ended up landing on it instead. Now this big DUMB FISH is stuck on the dock. He's HUNGRY. He's thrashing back and forth, and he's FLOPPING his tiny WILLY all around.
        vi. **MNEMONIC IMAGE**: www.pbrlinks.com/PRADERWILLI3

1. **KEY:** FISH represents the mode of diagnosis, HUGE/OBESE represents obesity, DUMB represents mental retardation, HUNGRY represents the insatiable appetite, and FLOPPING represents the hypotonia. In this mnemonic, you could also make Willy's eyes almond shaped and imagine that he has small fins.

21. The answer is C, "*Refer to urology for surgical correction*" Most cases of hypospadias do require repair. There are several reasons for this, including cosmetic appearance, proper growth of penis, ability for a male to urinate while standing and self-esteem. A circumcision should be postponed in all children with hypospadias because the foreskin is often used during the repair.

22. The answer is B, "*Prune Belly Syndrome*" The patient has PRUNE BELLY SYNDROME. This should be considered in any child with **urinary tract abnormalities and cryptorchidism (absent testicles in the scrotum) or undescended testicles**. Look for the other cardinal sign of **weak abdominal musculature** due to deficient abdominal muscles. The urinary tract anomalies include vesico**ureter**al reflux (VUR), posterior urethral valves (PUV) and renal dysplasia. The renal anomalies often result in **hydronephrosis, oligo**hydramnios and pulmonary hypoplasia. Children have a poor prognosis and many unfortunately die within a few months.

    a. PEARL: Look for a **newborn** with weak abdominal muscles, "undescended testes" (may actually be missing) and a midline abdominal mass (distended bladder or hydronephrosis).

23. The answer is C, "*Microcolon*" The image shows what is clearly a barium enema with a small caliber colon (think colon). This child has **megacystis microcolon intestinal hypoperistalsis syndrome**. It usually occurs in females and is associated with constipation, meconium ileus and urinary retention. The key to answering the question is to know what a normal colon should look like on a contrast study. This one is too thin.

    a. PEARL: **Hypoplastic left colon** is a condition that has a strong association with maternal diabetes (IDDM). Look for a colon that is small from the splenic flexure to the anus

24. The answer is A, "*ABO incompatibility*" The child has hyperbilirubinemia, and multiple possible reasons for hemolysis. Not that this is a FIRST-TIME pregnancy, which rules out Rhesus disease as a possible answer. Rh disease occurs during second pregnancies when immunoglobulins have formed against the Rh+ blood cells from a previous exposure. Also, ABO incompatibility tends to be associated with spherocytes, while Rh disease tends to be associated with nucleated RBCs (erythroblasts).

    a. PEARL: Hereditary spherocytosis can also result in hemolysis and jaundice, but you would **have to** be given "**SPLENOMEGALY**" as an exam finding.

    b. PEARL: If they refer to an RBC that does not have central pallor, they are referring to spherocytes.

QUESTIONS

25. (Multipart Question) A 16-year old girl presents to your office. She has never had a menstrual cycle. On physical exam she has stage 5 breasts and no pubic hair. Her BMI is 22. What's the diagnosis?
    a. Anorexia induced amenorrhea
    b. Turner Syndrome
    c. Androgen insensitivity
    d. Delayed puberty

26. (Multipart Question) For the patient in the previous question, what is the next best diagnostic test?
    a. Electrolyte panel
    b. Karyotype
    c. Luteinizing hormone
    d. Testosterone level

27. A 4-month old child present due to morning irritability. He has not had a feeding in 5 hours and is again quite irritable. A glucometer reading shows a glucose level of 46. You send stat labs and ask the mother to start feeding the child. Lactic acid level is elevated, ammonia level is normal and the anion gap is 16. Which of the following does the child have?
    a. Glycogen Storage Disease Type I (AKA von Gierke disease)
    b. Glycogen Storage Disease Type II (AKA Pompe disease)
    c. Niemann-Pick Disease
    d. Isovaleric Acidemia

28. (Multipart Question) A 4-year old child presents with a history of developmental delay. There has been concern that he may have autism. On exam you note that he has very light-colored skin, light-colored hair and a rash that appears eczematous. The mother says that he also tends to have "body odor." You note a musty or "mousy" odor. You send off a panel of labs and note that his glucose, ammonia, anion gap and lactic acid levels are all essentially normal. What's the diagnosis?
    a. Alkaptonuria
    b. Maple Syrup Urine Disease (MSUD)
    c. Homocysteinuria
    d. Phenylketonuria

29. (Multipart Question) The patient above is eventually diagnosed with an amino acid problem. What type of diet should be prescribed?
    a. A diet high in carbohydrates and fats but low in protein
    b. A diet that is low in the amino acid causing the problem
    c. A diet with that contains none of the amino acid causing the problem
    d. A diet that is high in carnitine

30. Infants born to diabetic mothers are at higher risk for all of the following EXCEPT:
    a. Hyperbilirubinemia
    b. Hypertrophic cardiomyopathy
    c. Hypoplastic left colon
    d. Sepsis

31. (MULTIPART QUESTION) A new rapid flu test has been released. You perform a study to compare results of the rapid test to those of influenza PCR testing. 120 patients were tested. 90 patients were confirmed to have the flu using PCR. Of those 90 patients, only 80 patients tested positive using the rapid test. Of the 30 patients confirmed by PCR to be negative for influenza, 5 patients tested positive by the new rapid test. What is the SENSITIVITY of the new rapid test?
    a. 71%
    b. 83%
    c. 89%
    d. 94%

32. (MULTIPART QUESTION) In the above study, what is the SPECIFICITY of the new rapid test?
    a. 71%
    b. 83%
    c. 89%
    d. 94%

33. (MULTIPART QUESTION) In the above study, what was the Positive Predictive Value of the new rapid test in the population that was tested?
    a. 71%
    b. 83%
    c. 89%
    d. 94%

34. A child presents with a history of mild mental retardation and hypercalcemia. On exam he is quite talkative, has a smooth philtrum, a broad nasal bridge, an elf-like face and a murmur. What's the most likely diagnosis?
    a. Fetal Alcohol Syndrome
    b. Williams Syndrome
    c. Down Syndrome
    d. Congenital Hyperparathyroidism

ANSWERS

25. The answer is C, "*Androgen insensitivity*" It's NOT A GENETIC FEMALE! Primary amenorrhea + breasts + **lack of pubic hair** = androgen insensitivity (AKA testicular feminization)!
    a. PEARL: Making the association between ANDROGENS and PUBIC hair is extremely important and very high yield.

26. The answer is B, "*Karyotype*" A karyotype will show that the patient has an XY genotype. The child was supposed to be a male, but due to defective androgen receptors, the "default" phenotype was created. Androgens are required for pubic hair, which is why this patent has none. Luteinizing hormone is a good screening test for PCOS.

27. The answer is A, "*Glycogen Storage Disease Type I (AKA von Gierke disease)*" GSD I is due to the inability use glycogen due to problems metabolizing glucose 6-phosphate (G6P). While patients can metabolize glucose itself and can break down glycogen, they are unable convert to glucose the G6P produced from glycogen or gluconeogenesis. In the less common variant, they are unable to transport the G6P. During fasting, there is hypoglycemia plus the buildup of glycogen, lactic acid and lipids as G6P is shunted to different reactions. Glycogen can build up in organs and cause organomegaly. The main treatment is to provide a constant source of glucose by giving starch. G6P key features: **hepatomegaly, hypoglycemia.**

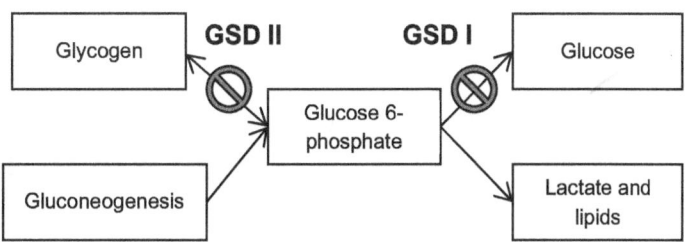

In **GSD II** (Pompe disease, lysosomal acid maltase deficiency), glycogen *cannot* be broken down in lysosomes, so accumulates in cells. It is a LYsosomal storage disorder that usually results in early cardiomyopathy with a large PUMP (heart), hence the mnemonics "PUMP-E's" and pompLay (lysosomal).

Niemann-Pick Disease is a sphingomyelinase deficiency that results in neurologic issues.
    a. PEARL: GSD I may present in babies when meals/feedings are starting to be spaced out. Also, for any patient presenting with morning issues, consider hypoglycemia as a possible reason.
    b. PEARL: HOT, HOT, HOT TOPIC! The Inborn Errors Of Metabolism Chapter is very high-yield, but tends to be very difficult to master. If you are short on time, just memorize the summary table and focus on the rest of the core study guide since other topics are going to be more easily memorized/learned.

28. The answer is D, "*Phenylketonuria*" Aminoacidopathies are disorders in which isolated amino acids cannot be broken down. Since the problem is limited to only a particular amino acid, there is no significant elevation in ammonia levels (the exception is maple syrup urine disease, MSUD). Also, there is no acidosis because this is not a fuel issue (carbohydrate and fat metabolism are working fine, but once again MSUD is the exception). The disorders include phenylketonuria (PKU), alkaptonuria, MSUD, homocystinuria and tyrosinemia.

29. The answer is B, "*A diet that is low in the amino acid causing the problem*" PHENYLKETONURIA (PKU) is a deficiency of phenylalanine hydroxylase. Phenylalanine can't be broken down into tyrosine. If left untreated, patients will be asymptomatic for a few months. They can then start to present with developmental delay, a musty/mousy odor, skin/hair changes (LIGHT colored skin and hair; possibly eczema-like rash) and eventually might even carry a diagnosis of "autism" because of severe mental retardation. The disease is also associated with septal defects.

    All states test for this on the newborn screen, which looks for an elevated phenylalanine level. Your first step in neonates should be to REPEAT the test because some kids have a TRANSIENT elevation in their phenylalanine level at birth. If it's abnormal again, the child still might be ok because it may just be that the enzyme hasn't matured yet. Consult a geneticist to sort it out. The goal should be to start treatment by 14 days of life, otherwise severe mental retardation can occur.

    TYROSINE levels will be low or nonexistent in kids with PKU, so tyrosine becomes an essential amino acid. Some children require tyrosine supplementation in the diet. The general treatment, though, is a LOW PHENYLALANINE DIET. OVER-TREATING (meaning zero phenylalanine) can result in lethargy, rash and diarrhea (don't get it confused with pellagra!). Also, if an affected pregnant mother has poor dietary control, her child can be born with microcephaly, congenital heart defects (CHD) and cognitive defects.

    a. PEARL: Look for a child that looks like they might have albinism. Also, keep in mind that the newborn screen is only valid AFTER protein intake.
    b. MNEMONIC: Imagine walking into a smelly basement. You say, "PEE-YEW!" Just then you see a LIGHT-SKINNED MOUSE with WHITE HAIR running by. You scream, "EEW," and run away.
        - KEY: PEE-YEW = PKU. LIGHT COLORS = Light skin and hair. EEW = PKU again. You could consider adding a TYRE (for tyrosine) to the story, and imagine that the mouse runs out of an old tire in the corner.

30. The answer is D, "*Sepsis*" For the ABP exam, an infant of a diabetic mother (IDM) is at higher risk for congenital heart disease, congenital heart disease and CHD! Patients are especially prone to having septal defects. May also have coarctation of the aorta, hypertrophic obstructive cardiomyopathy (HOCM), truncus arteriosus, dextrocardia and more. Can also have rib or vertebral column abnormalities, hydrocephalus, macrosomia/LGA size (with birth trauma), small left colon, duodenal atresia (double bubble... or "gaseous distention in both the stomach and duodenum"), apnea, hypOcalcemia, hypOmagnesemia, hypOphosphatemia, hyperbilirubinemia, polycythemia, vascular thromboses and RDS (look for tachypnea). Surprisingly, sepsis is not more common in an IDM.

    a. PEARL: The hypoglycemia may not occur until ONE or TWO days after birth.
    b. PEARL: For hypocalcemia, look for jitteriness, a prolonged QT, Chvostek's sign (tapping the facial nerve elicits a twitch) or Trousseau's sign (carpopedal spasm noted when the wrist is clasped).

31. The answer is C, "*89%*"

32. The answer is B, "*83%*"

33. The answer is D, "94%"

   a. **STATISTICS OVERVIEW**: Some of these can be quick and easy "give me" points on the exam if you know where to put in the numbers and how to use the formulas. Please MEMORIZE the table below. TP & TN = True Positives & True Negatives. FP & FN = False Positives & False Negatives. PPV & NPV = Positive Predictive Value & Negative Predictive Value. In the PBR Core Study Guide, **the "validity hierarchy" of different types of research studies is discussed**. This was added to PBR based on repeated requests from past PBR members. The boards could ask you which type of study design has higher validity, or you may be asked to choose the best type of study for a particular problem being researched. MAKE SURE you go through that material in the Core Study Guide!

   TP & TN = True Positives & True Negatives. FP & FN = False Positives & False Negatives. PPV & NPV = Positive Predictive Value & Negative Predictive Value.

	DISEASE (+)	DISEASE (-)	
TEST (+)	TP:	FP:	PPV = TP/(TP+FP) = Proportional to Prevalence
TEST (-)	FN:	TN:	NPV = TN/(TN+FN) = Not Proportional to Prevalence (Inversely Proportional to Prevalence)
	SENSITIVITY = TP/(TP+FN)	SPECIFICITY = TN/(TN+FP)	THIS BLOCK = TOTAL # OF PATIENTS STUDIED = ROW TOTAL = COLUMN TOTAL

   b. **PEARLS/MNEMONICS**: Note that everything you need to calculate is ALWAYS in either one **column** or **row**. Also, letters are bolded as a memory aid. N-P-N-P (se**N**sitivity, s**P**ecificity, **N**pv, **P**pv).

   c. For the questions asked, the table should have looked something like this

	DISEASE (+)	DISEASE (-)	TOTAL	
TEST (+)	TP: 80	FP: 5	85	PPV: 80/85 = **94%**
TEST (-)	FN: 10	TN: 25	35	NPV: 25/35 = **71%**
TOTAL	90	30	120	
	SENSITIVITY: 80/90 = **89%**	SPECIFICITY: 25/30 = **83%**		

   d. TERMINOLOGY:

- SENSITIVITY = TP/(TP+FN). A high sensitivity [TP/(TP+FN)] is needed for SCREENING tests in order to rule out the presence of disease in a healthy patient. These are tests that are being done to RULE OUT a disease. So, a screening test should have a high sensitivity, which will mean that a negative result rules out the disease in that patient.
    - **MNEMONIC**: sp**IN** & sn**OUT**. sn**OUT** should remind you that Se**N**sitivity (**SN**out) is related to ruling **OUT** a disease.
- SPECIFICITY = TN/(TN+FP). A high specificity [TN/(TN+FP)] is needed for CONFIRMATORY tests. These are tests that are done to RULE IN (AKA CONFIRM) a disease. So, a confirmatory test should have a high specificity, which will mean that a positive result rules in the disease in that patient.
    - **MNEMONIC**: sp**IN** & sn**OUT**. sp**IN** should remind you that **SP**ecificity (**SP**in) is related to ruling **IN** a disease.
- POSITIVE PREDICTIVE VALUE = TP/(TP+FP). The positive predictive value [TP/(TP+FP)] looks at all of the POSITIVE results from a test and predicts how likely it is that a positive result actually means a patient has the disease. For example, what are the chances that a patient with a positive flu test actually has the flu? The positive predictive value of a test depends on how prevalent it is in the population being tested. Think about it: even given the same sensitivity and specificity, a positive test for influenza is more likely to indicate true disease than is a positive test for smallpox, since smallpox has a prevalence of zero.
- NEGATIVE PREDICTIVE VALUE = TN/(TN+FN). The negative predictive value [TN/(TN+FN)] looks at all of the NEGATIVE results from a test and predicts how likely it is that a negative result actually means a patient does not have the disease. For example, what are the chances that a patient with a negative flu test in fact does not have the flu? As with PPV, NPV depends on prevalence, but inversely.
- NULL HYPOTHESIS: The null hypothesis is stated at the beginning of a research study. It assumes that the outcome being studied is the result of pure chance. In other words, it assumes that there is no variable (environmental exposure, medication, etc.) that could result in an increase in this outcome. For example, if studying the association between smoking and lung cancer, the null hypothesis would state that there is no increase in lung cancer in patients who smoke.
- P VALUE: The P value represents the chance that the null hypothesis would be rejected if it were actually true. In other words, what is the chance that a true null hypothesis would be accidentally rejected? Or, what would be the chance of the observed results if there were no true difference?
- SIGNIFICANT RESULTS: Results of a study are considered significant if the P value is **< 0.05**. They are considered "highly significant" if the P value is < 0.01. Note that statistical significance is not related to clinical significance; a finding that is highly significant statistically simply means that it is very unlikely to have occurred by chance, not that it matters clinically.
- TYPE I ERROR: Type I errors basically mean that a study claimed there was a significant difference when there in fact was not one.
    - **MNEMONIC**: Type "i" error. I made the error and said this is the greatest test on earth when I shouldn't have. Or, i claimed fame for discovering an association

between patients born in December and a higher incidence of cancer. Turns out "i" just read the data wrong and made a type "i" error.

- **TYPE II ERROR:** Type II errors basically mean that a study claimed there was NO significant difference in the results when there in fact **was** one.
    - **MNEMONIC:** TWO rhymes with YOU. In a type TWO error, YOU made the mistake of claiming that my test or medicine doesn't work, when in fact it does! Think of it as a competition between two drug companies.
- **PREVALENCE:** Refers to the proportion of a population found to have a condition at a given point in time.
- **INCIDENCE:** This refers the number of new cases in a population over a given **period of time**. For example, if there were 30 new cases in a population of 2000 people over 2 years, that would equal 7.5 cases per 1000 person-years.
- **STATISTICAL POWER:** The ability of a test or study to find a true effect and avoid type II errors. Increasing the number of subjects always makes it easier to find true effects, but using the proper experimental design and statistical techniques can be equally important.
- **SAMPLE SIZE:** The number of subjects being studied. A larger sample size will increase statistical power and increase the ability of a study to detect adverse events.

34. The answer is B, "*Williams Syndrome*" (AKA WILLIAM'S SYNDROME): Though patients usually have mild mental retardation, they also tend to have relatively high verbal skills and a fun, "cocktail party" personality, so they get along great with other people. Facial features include an elf-like face ("ELFIN" FACE), a low and flat nasal bridge, an upturned nose, a smooth philtrum and wide-spaced teeth. Other problems include SUPRAvalvular aortic stenosis (not involving the valve, but the aorta itself), peripheral pulmonic stenosis and hypercalcemia. Then can occasionally also have hypothyroidism.

    a. PEARL: If you see the word SUPRAvalvular stenosis, have a HIGH suspicion for this diagnosis.
    b. IMAGE: www.pbrlinks.com/QA34A
    c. IMAGE: www.pbrlinks.com/QA34B
    d. MNEMONIC: Think of your favorite (or least favorite) celeb with the last name Williams for this mnemonic. Serena Williams? Robbie Williams? Robin Williams? Vanessa Williams? Now, imagine _____ WILLIAMS at a PARTY riding a COW around the PERIPHERY of the group. The cow has an ELFIN FACE and WIDELY SPACED TEETH. WILLIAMS is having fun, but ISN'T TOO SMART. S/he tries to make the cow go fast and then JUMP OVER A HURDLE. The COW suddenly stops and _____ WILLIAMS goes flying off the COW. S/he flies OVER THE HURDLE, and as s/he lands his/her PHILTRUM hits a rock. WILLIAMS' PHILTRUM is now LONG and the nose is UPTURNED. Now WILLIAMS is in the middle with the group on the PERIPHERY taking care of him/her.
    e. KEY: PARTY represents the personality, COW represents calcium for dairy products, PERIPHERY represents peripheral pulmonic stenosis, ISN'T TOO SMART represents the mild mental retardation and JUMP OVER THE HURDLE represents supravalvular stenosis (if you remember nothing else, remember THIS finding).

QUESTIONS

35. Patients with Alagille Syndrome are most likely to have problems with which of the following organ systems:
    a. Hepatic
    b. Neurologic
    c. Renal
    d. Respiratory

36. A child is born to a mother with a history of hyperparathyroidism. The child is predisposed to having which of the following:
    a. Hypercalcemia
    b. Hypocalcemia
    c. Hypophosphatemia
    d. None of the above.

37. A 4-month old had a prolonged seizure 6 days after his 2-month well child visit. He received the standard 2-month vaccinations. He now returns for his 4-month visit. Which of the following statements is true regarding DTaP?
    a. The child should no longer receive DTaP or any component of it ever again.
    b. The child should no longer receive DTaP, but may receive the aP component at this visit.
    c. The child should no longer receive DTaP, but may receive the DT component at this visit.
    d. The child may receive DTaP at this visit.
    e. The child should undergo allergy testing with the individual components.

38. Which of the following congenital infections is associated with nasal perforation?
    a. Toxoplasmosis
    b. Rubella
    c. Cytomegalovirus
    d. Herpes simplex
    e. Syphilis

39. A healthy-appearing child is born to a mother that had poor prenatal care. Late in her pregnancy, she was found to have syphilis that was confirmed with a positive FTA. She was treated with erythromycin 6 weeks prior to the delivery. Non-treponemal titers are obtained from both the mother and the neonate. Both are positive. What's the next best step in management?

    a. Treat the mother and the baby with penicillin.
    b. Treat the mother with penicillin and check the FTA in the baby.
    c. Do not treat the mother. Treat the baby with penicillin.
    d. Recheck the baby's non-treponemal titers in one month.

40. A 4-month old female is brought to an urgent care center. The mother is concerned about possible bleeding and is worried about a pink spot in the diaper. She brought the diaper to the visit, and upon inspection you clearly note a salmon-colored spot in the diaper. On physical examination, the child is healthy-appearing. Conjunctivae are pink. There is no blood noted at the vaginal introitus. Growth parameters are all at the 50th percentile, the child has a healthy appetite and breastfeeds well. A urine dip-stick shows no blood. What is the likely etiology?

    a. Vaginal spotting
    b. Nephrolithiasis
    c. Oxalate crystals
    d. Urate crystals

41. (Multipart Question) A 10-year old girl presents with a painful lump on her neck. She says the pain started about a week ago. On exam, you note a tender cervical lymph node that measures approximately 2.5 cm. She has no fever and the lesion is not draining. She has a cat at home but denies ever being scratched. What is the most likely etiology?

    a. Staphylococcus aureus
    b. Streptococcus pyogenes
    c. Streptococcus pneumoniae
    d. Bartonella henselae
    e. Atypical mycobacteria

42. (Multipart Question) What is the next best step in management for the above patient?

    a. Incision and drainage
    b. Obtain a biopsy and send for pathology and culture
    c. Treat with amoxicillin-clavulanate
    d. Place a PPD
    e. Watchful waiting with follow-up in 7 days

43. An infant is brought in for a well-child visit. She has been noted to cough with feeds, even more so since the introduction of solids. A barium swallow is shown with multiple images (www.pbrlinks.com/QA43A and www.pbrlinks.com/QA43B). What is the most likely diagnosis?

   a. Achalasia
   b. Tracheoesophageal fistula with a blind pouch
   c. H-type tracheoesophageal fistula
   d. Esophageal web
   e. Reflux

ANSWERS

35. The answer is A, "*Hepatic*" ALAGILLE SYNDROME (AKA ARTERIOHEPATIC DYSPLASIA, AKA ALLAGILE SYNDROME) is a genetic disorder in which jaundice is noted in the newborn period. Look for a child with LIVER and HEART disease. Here are some associations: **paucity of bile ducts (AKA intrahepatic biliary atresia or hypoplastic biliary ducts), pulmonary stenosis, a triangular face** (underdeveloped mandible), hypercholesterolemia with xanthomas, eye abnormalities and acholic stools.

    a. IMAGE: www.pbrlinks.com/QA35A

    b. MNEMONIC IMAGES:

      - MNEMONIC IMAGE #1: The GREEN ALLIGATOR has a TRIANGULAR FACE that is green because it is filled with BILE. His head is shaped like a HEART to remind of the PULMONARY STENOSIS. He also has funny shaped EYES and XANTHOMATOUS lumps all over his face. Also, notice what he's eating. It's a LIVER!

      - MNEMONIC IMAGE #2: This cute little guy is named Alagille. He has a TRIANGULAR head and a funny shaped JAW that is in the shape of a HEART to remind you of PULMONARY STENOSIS.

      - MNEMONIC IMAGE #3: That's Al the Green Alligator.

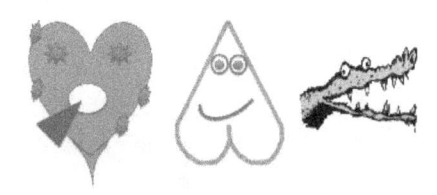

36. The answer is B, "*Hypocalcemia*" HYPOCALCEMIA (Ca **< 8.5**, or ionized Ca **<4.5**): This is less common than **hyper**calcemia, but has much greater morbidity associated with it and is thus more heavily tested on the boards. Can range from minimal symptoms due to mild hypocalcemia from hyperventilation to HORRIBLE outcomes. Symptoms of hypocalcemia include: **paresthesias, tetany**, carpopedal spasm/tetany (also known as **Trousseau's sign**), **Chvostek's sign** (abnormal reaction/tetany of the facial nerve when tapped), Seizures that do not respond to benzodiazepines, laryngospasm (resulting in tachypnea; can look/sound like croup), **prolonged QT**.

    a. MNEMONICS:

      - Carpopedal spasm due to hypocalcemia = Trousseau's sign = "TROUSER'S" Sign = Think of it affecting the extremities!

      - **CH**eeky **CH**vostek sign!

      - Paresthesias and muscle spasms: Most of us have had an anxious patient in the emergency room who complains of transient numbness and tingling in their hands and/or feet; it's due to transient hypocalcemia from hyperventilation. If you can remember this association, you can remember that all of these tetany-like symptoms are related to hypOcaclemia!

    b. EARLY HYPOCALCEMIA: Occurring within the first 3 days of life. Differential includes INFANT OF A DIABETIC MOTHER, MATERNAL HYPERPARATHYROIDISM, ASPHYXIA and IUGR

    c. LATE HYPOCALCEMIA: Occurring after DOL 7. Much wider differential, including:

- HYPOMAGNESEMIA: Hypomagnesemia causes PTH resistance and decreased PTH secretion, which in turn cause hypocalcemia. May not respond to the calcium gluconate.
    - (DOUBLE TAKE) PEARLS: **Magnesium sulfate infusion** (for tocolysis or preeclampsia) can result in severe hypocalcemia and possible hypomagnesemia. The mechanism is complex/unknown. Treat with calcium gluconate, but keep in mind that patients may not respond as quickly as would normally be expected. So if you are given a vignette about a hypocalcemic baby not responding to calcium gluconate, consider magnesium tocolysis as the etiology.
- DIGEORGE SYNDROME (22Q11 DELETION): Parathyroid problems resulting in low calcium, velocardiofacial defects, etc.
- HYPOPARATHYROIDISM: low calcium, high phosphorus
- PSEUDOHYPOPARATHYROIDISM: Autosomal dominant disorder resulting in resistance to PTH. Therefore, serum PTH will be **high but serum calcium will be low and phosphorus will be high!** This is a "pseudo" disorder but the clinical effects are real. Look for short/stubby 4th digits (fingers and/or toes), developmental delay, obesity, and moon facies.
- VITAMIN D DEFICIENCY: Decreased calcium absorption
- ALKALOSIS: Shifts ionized/active calcium to the protein-bound form.
- ETHYLENE GLYCOL POISONING:
    - MNEMONIC: Calcium oxalate crystals (shaped like long beer cans, or needles) are found in the urine with ethylene glycol, so just assume that there is SOO much calcium lost in the urine during this process that it results in hypocalcemia! Remember, the calcium oxalate crystals that have the X on them are unrelated.
- RHABDOMYOLYSIS: Calcium deposition into the muscles results in intravascular hypocalcemia.
- RENAL FAILURE: Results in an inability to hydroxylate Vitamin D to 1,25 form.
- NEPHROTIC SYNDROME: There is low albumin, so the measured albumin-bound calcium level is also low. Check the ionized calcium level.

37. The answer is C, "*The child should no longer receive DTaP, but may receive the DT component at this visit.*" **DTaP CONTRAINDICATIONS**: ENCEPHALOPATHY or "PROLONGED" SEIZURE should trigger an alert! If a child has **encephalopathy** or a **"prolonged" seizure within 1 week** of getting DTaP, the **PERTUSSIS (aP)** component is contraindicated in future vaccinations. Instead, **give DT**. Please remember that this is possibly a reaction to the PERTUSSIS component, and not the tetanus component. Also, DO NOT order allergy testing because you may induce a seizure!
    a. PROGRESSIVE NEUROLOGIC DISORDER: If a child has a neurologic disorder that is considered progressive, or has a seizure disorder that is not yet under control, then DTaP is **relatively** contraindicated. If the neurologic disorder has been stabilized or is no longer progressive, you MAY give DTaP.
    b. OTHER **RELATIVE** CONTRAINDICATIONS: Having a **brief** seizure within 3 days, a high fever (>105°) within 48 hours, or a shock-like state within 48 hours of previous administration.
        - PEARL/MNEMONIC: If tested on one of these 3 *relative* contraindications You are more likely to be given a case in which the child had an issue 4-7 days from the date of previous

vaccination. This would make the answer clear (give DTaP!). Therefore, keeping the FOURTH day in mind as the day when the child is in the clear might help with these 3 relative contraindications.

38. The answer is E, "*Syphilis*" Syphilis is associated with a maculopapular rash, hepatosplenomegaly, **PEELING SKIN, PERFORATED NASAL SEPTUM** and **HUTCHINSON TEETH.**

39. The answer is C, "*Do not treat the mother. Treat the baby with penicillin.*" If mom was given **ERYTHROMYCIN**, as in the scenario presented, TREAT the baby because erythromycin doesn't cross the placenta. Penicillin is the best treatment for syphilis and WILL cross the placenta and will therefore treat both MOM and BABY. Syphilis is caused by TREPONEMA PALLIDUM. Non-treponemal tests (RPR or VDRL) can be FALSE positives, so you need to do a confirmatory treponemal test (FTA). While the FTA does not correlate with disease activity, the non-treponemal tests do. Also, the non-treponemal tests may eventually disappear with decreased disease activity. So once disease presence is confirmed with FTA, look at disease activity with non-treponemal titers to help guide management. Neonates born to a mother with a reactive non-treponemal (RPR or VDRL) test result should have a quantitative non-treponemal serologic test (RPR or VDRL) performed on the infant's serum. Treponemal serologic tests (FTA) on a baby are difficult to interpret so are not recommended. An immunoglobulin (IgM) test is also not currently available. If the mom was treated and the baby's titers are lower than hers, it's safe to assume that those are just the mom's IgGs that crossed the placenta and that there is NO NEED TO TREAT (just follow the titers). If the mom was treated < 1 month ago, TREAT. If the mom was given Erythromycin, TREAT because it doesn't cross the placenta.

    a. CONGENITAL SYPHILIS: Baby born with maculopapular rash, HSM, **PEELING SKIN, PERFORATED NASAL SEPTUM** or **HUTCHINSON TEETH**. These teeth are peg-shaped (cone-like) teeth but also have a **central notch** that is extremely specific for congenital syphilis. Treat with PENICILLIN.

    b. CONDYLOMA LATA: Refers to SECONDARY SYPHILIS, in which white-gray coalescing papules are seen.

    c. PEARLS:
       - If the FTA is positive but VDRL is negative, also consider LYME DISEASE (BORRELIA BURGDORFERI).
       - NAME ALERT/MNEMONIC: Condyloma LATA (AKA "condyloma FLATa," are much more FLAT than Condyloma ACUMINATA ("accumulated"; found with HPV infections).
       - NAME ALERT/MNEMONIC: Peg teeth are also found in patients with Incontinentia Pigmenti (AKA "Incontinentia PEGmentia")
       - IMAGE (PEG-SHAPED TEETH): www.pbrlinks.com/QA39A
       - IMAGE (HUTCHINSON TEETH): www.pbrlinks.com/QA39B

40. The Answer is D, "*Urate crystals*" **URIC ACID CRYSTALS: Seen in breast-fed babies and is harmless!** It can also be associated with rapid cell turnover and hyperuricemia (as seen in lymphomas).

    a. PEARL: Look for a breast fed baby presenting with a pink spot in the diaper! Uric acid turns to a salmon or pink colored powder when it dries. It scares parents to heck, but only requires reassurance.

    b. IMAGE: www.pbrlinks.com/QA40A

41. The answer is B, "*Streptococcus pyogenes*"

42. The answer is C, *"Treat with amoxicillin-clavulanate"* This is ACUTE and TENDER lymphadenopathy (< 3 weeks) in the neck area. Bartonella and atypical mycobacteria tend to cause CHRONIC lymphadenopathy. STREPTOCOCCUS PYOGENES (AKA GAS or STREP PYOGENES) is your most likely culprit. Next in line is Staph aureus, especially if it's in a neonate, or if it's an acute lymphadenopathy associated with drainage of purulent material. Know the difference between the different types of Streptococcal species, as well as the different presentations for Staph versus Strep. You should also be familiar with the differential diagnosis of tender versus non-tender lymphadenopathy. Here is an excerpt from the core study guide on the differential for acute lymphadenopathy (refer to the study guide for more in-depth discussion):

    a. STAPH: Look for cervical or submandibular lymphadenopathy in a neonate or infant. May also present as a breast abscess.

    - PEARLS: This is one of the few circumstances in which you would choose Staph as the correct answer if presented with a neonate. Also, while GBS is a common answer for neonates, GROUP A STREP (AKA GAS or Strep pyogenes) is probably NEVER the answer for a neonate.

    b. GROUP A STREP (GAS or STREP PYOGENES): Look for an **older child** with **impetigo**, **pharyngitis** or even a single inflamed **lymph node**.

    c. PREAURICULAR LYMPHADENOPATHY: Consider adenovirus if you see a patient with conjunctivitis. Mononucleosis may present with acute or chronic lymphadenopathy.

    d. EMPIRIC TREATMENT: Aim to cover beta-lactamase producers. AMOXICILLIN-CLAVULANATE! Other appropriate options include cefazolin, clindamycin and erythromycin.

43. The answer is D, *"Esophageal web"* An ESOPHAGEAL WEB can cause reflux-like symptoms, esophageal impaction and chest pain. It results from the failure of the esophagus to re-canalize in utero. The web then acts as an obstruction to the passage of a food bolus. Liquids, however, pass through more easily. Treatment requires dilation of the esophageal web.

    a. IMAGES: www.pbrlinks.com/QA43A and www.pbrlinks.com/QA43B

    - PEARL: The "jet phenomenon" can make certain images look like a TE fistula.

    b. TRACHEOESOPHAGEAL FISTULA: There are several types of tracheoesophageal fistulas. For the commonly tested H-type TE fistula, look for increased coughing with liquids as they seep through the fistula and enter the trachea. A TE fistula with a blind esophageal pouch is the most common type of TE fistula. More specifically, the upper part of the esophagus is a blind pouch, and the lower part connects with the trachea.

    - PEARL: H-type TE fistulas may be discovered after a newborn leaves the hospital. The other two will surely be found prior to discharge. Look for a blind pouch on a barium swallow, a history of polyhydramnios, symptoms consistent with VACTERL or an image showing a curled nasogastric tube. For an H-type fistula, you could be given a history that is consistent with the fistula and an image showing a nasogastric tube going all the way to the stomach.

    c. ACHALASIA: Associated with forceful vomiting.

QUESTIONS

44. A 9-month old child presents for routine follow-up. The child is healthy-appearing. The mother gives the infant to you for your exam. During the exam, the infant seems anxious, begins to cry, then stops breathing, becomes unresponsive and has some jerking movements. The pulse is measured at approximately 70 beats per minute. What's the best next step in management?

    a. Activate EMS and begin CPR
    b. Provide positive pressure ventilation
    c. Provide oxygen by nasal cannula
    d. Blow on the face
    e. Observe

45. An LGA baby is born after a difficult breech delivery. The patient is noted have tachypnea. A chest X-ray is obtained and it shows unilateral diaphragmatic elevation. What is the likely etiology?

    a. Abdominal trauma with hematoma
    b. Asphyxia
    c. Erb's Palsy
    d. Klumpke Palsy

46. What type of hearing screen is recommended in a 4-month old child?

    a. Automated auditory brainstem response
    b. Otoacoustic emissions
    c. Visual reinforced audiometry
    d. Pure tone audiometry

47. What type of hearing screen is recommended in a 6-year old child?

    a. Automated auditory brainstem response
    b. Otoacoustic emissions
    c. Visual reinforced audiometry
    d. Pure tone audiometry

48. A girl in college is brought to the ER. She is confused, hyperthermic, and with red colored urine. Her roommate states that she went to a party on the previous night. What is the likely etiology?

    a. Heroin related reaction
    b. Lysergic acid diethylamide (LSD)-related reaction
    c. Ecstasy related reaction
    d. Alcohol dehydrogenase deficiency

49. Name the inheritance pattern the following image most likely represents:

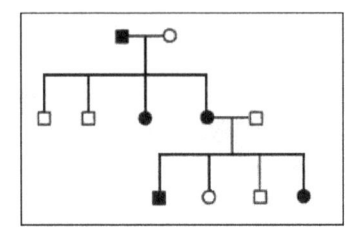

    a. Autosomal dominant
    b. Autosomal recessive
    c. X-linked dominant
    d. X-linked recessive

50. A 2-year old boy is brought to the ER. His patents entered his room last night and saw a bat. The child was sleeping quietly at the time. The parents tried to catch the bat, but it flew out of the window before they could do so. What is the next best step in management?

    a. Provide rabies vaccination
    b. Provide human rabies immunoglobulin (HRIG)
    c. Provide both rabies vaccination and human rabies immunoglobulin (HRIG)
    d. If a thorough physical exam reveals no bite marks, provide reassurance and discharge the patient.

ANSWERS

44. The answer is E, "*Observe*" The child had a BREATH-HOLDING SPELL. These are most common between **6 to 18** months of age. Children have **apneic episodes in response to pain, fear, anger, frustration or injury**. Children can become **unconscious** or even have a **seizure** with a postictal period. EEG is always normal. No specific treatment is required except making sure that children don't hurt themselves during a seizure. The two subtypes of breath holding spells include cyanotic breath holding (associated with anger, frustration, and cyanosis) and pallid breath holding (associated with fear, pain, injury and a pale or "pallid" appearance).

45. The answer is C, "*Erb's Palsy*" Both ERB'S PALSY and KLUMPKE PALSY are associated with birth trauma, BREECH delivery, caesarian sections, clavicle fractures and LGA births, but ERB's palsy is more likely to be associated with a **unilateral diaphragmatic paralysis**.

    a. PEARLS: **Images** of the arm/hand deformities MAY look the same. The only way to discern which palsy the child has is to evaluate the patient for specific neurologic limitations. If the baby is able to grasp, it is an ERB'S PALSY. If you note a claw hand deformity in a patient able to flex at the elbow, it is a KLUMPKE PALSY.

    b. ERBS PALSY (AKA ERB'S PALSY): Brachial plexus injury at C5-7 resulting in paralysis of the UPPER ARM. There is a "waiter's tip" configuration and **UNILATERAL DIAPHRAGMATIC PARALYSIS**.

        - IMAGE: www.pbrlinks.com/QA45A

        - PEARLS: The grasp and extension of the hand are INTACT. Respiratory distress can result due to phrenic nerve injury (look for a broken clavicle) resulting in unilateral diaphragmatic paralysis. Often associated with LGA babies, breech deliveries and C-sections.

        - MNEMONIC: Imagine a WAITER named "ERB" subtly asking for a tip. He CAN grasp the money you give to him.

    c. KLUMPKE PALSY: Brachial plexus injury, but lower (C7-T1). This affects the LOWER arm and hand. Worse prognosis because the nerves are typically torn. Results in a CLAW HAND deformity in which there is an INABILITY TO GRASP.

        - MNEMONIC: Hand is stuck in a configuration in which the hand has a KLUMP OF AIR in it.

46. The answer is A, "*Automated auditory brainstem response*" For details, please refer to the next answer.

47. The answer is D, "*Pure tone audiometry.*"

    a. SCREENING IN INFANTS < 6 MONTHS OLD: Use the ABR or OAE.

        - **AUTOMATED AUDITORY BRAINSTEM RESPONSE**: Measures brainstem response to sounds. This is better than the OAE test. It can check for unilateral, bilateral, conductive and/or sensory hearing loss. The infant **should be sleeping** for best results, therefore it is difficult to administer in children > 6-months of age.

        - **OTOACOUSTIC EMISSIONS TESTING**: This measures sounds that are made by the normally functioning cochlea in response to external sound. There is much more room for error in a noisy environment. Cost is similar, but false positives result in frequent audiology referrals. The infant **should be sleeping** for best results, therefore it is difficult to administer in children > 6-months of age.

b. SCREENING CHILDREN 6 MONTHS TO 2 YEARS OLD: For these preschoolers, use **VISUAL REINFORCED AUDIOMETRY**. This checks for bilateral hearing loss.

c. SCREENING CHILDREN OF SCHOOL AGE: Use **PURE TONE AUDIOMETRY**. At this age, children can wear headphones and let the examiner know which side the sound is coming from.

48. The answer is C, "*Ecstasy related reaction*" The patient in the vignette has malignant hyperthermia. This is an inherited disorder that can result in fever, confusion, muscle contractions and even rhabdomyolysis after exposure to a trigger such as anesthesia or a stimulant drug. Rhabdomyolysis can cause myoglobinuria (red or brown urine). She was likely exposed to ecstasy (AKA methylenedioxymethamphetamine and MDMA) the previous night. Ecstasy use is also associated with seizures, coma and short-term memory loss.

49. The answer is C, "*X-linked dominant.*" In an X-linked dominant disorder. Affected females may, or may not, pass on her defective X chromosome to their sons or daughters. There is **NEVER** male-to-male transmission AND there is **ALWAYS transmission of the disorder from an affected male to his daughters** (fathers will always pass on their defective X chromosome to their daughters). The latter point can help differentiate between an X-linked dominant and an autosomal dominant pedigree.

    a. PEARLS:

    - X-linked disorders are **RULED OUT** if you see male-to-male transmissions!

    - A vignette about a male patient that discusses ANYTHING about a MATERNAL UNCLE should alert you to possible X-linked disorder.

    - Most X-linked disorders are X-linked RECESSIVE. The dominant ones seem to select themselves out. These X-linked recessive disorders tend to be enzyme or protein deficiencies, thus several inborn errors of metabolism are X-linked recessive.

50. The answer is C, "*Provide both rabies vaccination and human rabies immunoglobulin (HRIG)*" RABIES is caused by a VIRAL infection transmitted through bites, scratches and contact with mucous membranes of infected animals, such as BATS, dogs, foxes, **RACCOONS** (most common in US), skunks, and WOODCHUCKS. If the history suggests a possible exposure (wild/aggressive animal), treat with standard wound care **PLUS** human rabies immunoglobulin (HRIG) **PLUS** the 4 vaccine doses. If the animal is a pet, observation of the patient and animal is allowed without giving HRIG.

    a. PEARL: Rabbits, rats and squirrels (rodents) are **NOT** associated with rabies.

    b. PEARL: For the boards, if the word "BAT" is mentioned (alive, escaped, whatever!), treat as an exposure!

Pediatrics Board Review

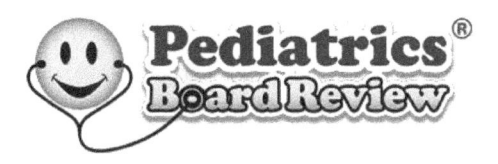

Hope You've Enjoyed It!
A Few [CRITICAL] Reminders

ARE YOU TAKING THE INITIAL CERTIFICATION EXAM? TAKE THE RISK CALCULATOR!

This exam is MUCH HARDER than the USMLE exams. In order to understand how many time you should go through the material, and in order to understand HOW to go through the material, you go through the **PBR RISK CALCULATOR** now and find out if you are at low, moderate or high risk of failing the exam. Then you'll know if you should go through the PBR Core Study Guide and the Q&A Book a minimum of 3 times or 5 times. **For low-risk test-takers**, AT LEAST 3 rounds of the material is recommended. **For high-risk test-takers**, AT LEAST 5 rounds of the material is recommended AND a strong focus on test-taking strategy. Your risk profile depends on many factors (e.g., exam history, scores on in-training exams, your residency program, and more). Visit www.pbrlinks.com/RISK-CALCULATOR and go through the **PBR RISK CALCULATOR** now.

"LOW-ISH" USMLE SCORES? FAILED A BOARD EXAM? WORK ON TECHNIQUE!

Seriously, seriously, SERIOUSLY! This exam can wreak havoc and chaos in you life. The techniques that are taught in PBR'S Test-Taking Strategies & Coaching courses have helped pediatricians finally pass the boards after they had failed MULTIPLE times. Learn the "board game" by understanding question-answering STRATEGIES. Start seeing an increase in your practice exam scores IMMEDIATELY. **PBR has helped a pediatrician pass on her 11th attempt!** So helping YOU should be easy. Don't have regrets. Visit the link below now and learn more about our self-paced and LIVE Test-Taking Strategies Courses. And if you're a high-risk test-taker, PLEASE consider signing up for the **VIP BUNDLE**.

www.pediatricsboardreview.com/**technique**

DON'T FORGET TO DO TONS OF BOARD REVIEW QUESTIONS... FOR PRACTICE!

Do at least 1000 practice questions if you're studying for the ABP initial certification boards, and at least 300 if you're taking the ABP MOC recertification exam. The first choice is the AAP PREP® series of questions, but PBR also has trusted affiliate relationships with other great companies that give you MASSIVE discounts on questions to use for PRACTICE! Just visit www.pediatricsboardreview.com/**tools** for member discounts.

MAXIMIZE YOUR LEARNING OPPORTUNITIES & MODALITIES!

PBR helps you **study EFFICIENTLY**. It's an entire SYSTEM that BUILDS on itself to give you the highest chance of passing your board exam. **REPETITION and MULTIMODAL** studying have both been **proven to increase learning**. The videos, the MP3s, and the summertime live webinars will help you **maximize your time and learning!** Visit www.pediatricsboardreview.com **now** and find the right PBR resource to help you maximize your learning efficiently (MP3s, Video Course, Webinars, Pediatric Atlas…).

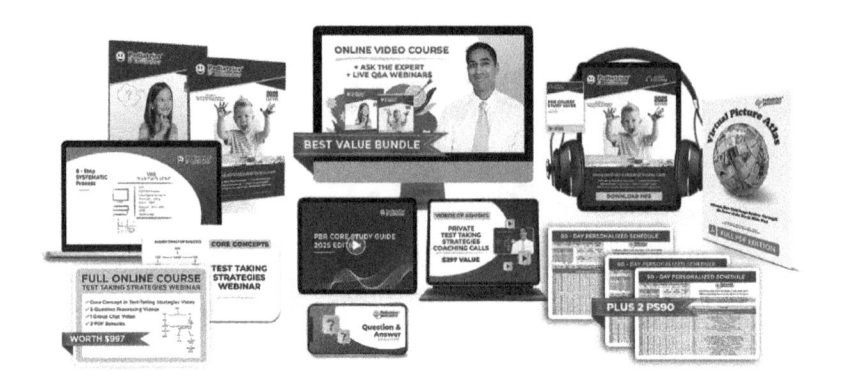

CAN'T DECIDE WHAT TO USE NEXT? YOU DON'T HAVE TO!

PBR is now offering a discounted bundle that includes **ALL OF OUR BOARD REVIEW products for over 50% off**. This should **remove the mental obstacles of money and finances** that sometimes causes pediatricians to fail. The package is called the **PBR No Brainer**, and it includes a video course, an audio course, live (and recorded) webinars, an online digital picture atlas, our hardcopy Core Study Guide, our hardcopy Q&A Book, our Full Online Test-Taking Strategies Course and evern a Personalized Study Schedule created just for you!

Visit the Link Below and Learn More About the **No Brainer** Enrollment & Upgrade Opportunities

www.pediatricsboardreview.com/no-brainer

ARE YOU GOING THROUGH MOCA-PEDS?

MOCA-Peds participants do NOT need the PBR Core Study Guide or the PBR Q&A Book. Instead, you need the (super cheap) **MOCA-PBR Study Guide & Test Companion** to help you quickly and EFFICIENTLY run through this year's 45 Learning Objectives and 3 Featured Readings. Then you can also use the MOCA-PBR as a "test-companion" on your "open book" and "open computer" MOCA-Peds questions. It's kind of amazing.

Visit www.pediatricsboardreview.com/MOCA-PBR and Learn More Now

ARE YOU TAKING THE TRADITIONAL, 4-HOUR MOC EXAM?

Going through the PBR Core Study Guide and Q&A Book 2 times should be PLENTY. The pass rate for the PBR has historically 100% for multiple years in a row for practicing general pediatricians. The most common feedback is along the lines of, "Ashish! I only read it once... and I passed!"

Again, CONGRATS on getting through this! Now let's do it again!!!

Ashish & Team PBR